Physical

BOARD REVIEW

Therapy

Physical

BOARD REVIEW

Therapy

Brad Fortinberry, DPT, SCS
St. Luke Home Health Agency
Bogue Chitto, MS

Michael Dunaway, PT
Staff Physical Therapist, Southwest Mississippi Regional Medical Center
Southwest Center for Rehabilitation, McComb, Mississippi

HANLEY & BELFUS, INC. / Philadelphia
An Imprint of Elsevier

Publisher: HANLEY & BELFUS, INC.
              Medical Publishers
              An Imprint of Elsevier
              210 South 13th Street
              Philadelphia, PA 19107
              (210) 546-7293; 800-962-1892
              Web site: http://www.hanleyandbelfus.com

Note to the reader: Although the information in this book has been carefully reviewed for correctness of dosage and indications, neither the authors nor the publisher can accept any legal responsibility for any errors or omissions that may be made. Neither the publisher nor authors make any warranty, expressed or implied, with respect to the material contained herein. Before prescribing any drug, the reader must review the manufacturer's current product information (package inserts) for accepted indications, absolute dosage recommendations, and other information pertinent to the safe and effective use of the product described. This is especially important when drugs are given in combination or as an adjunct to other forms of therapy.

ISBN-13: 978-1-56053-497-6
ISBN-10: 1-56053-497-4

Library of Congress Control Number: 2002104831

PHYSICAL THERAPY BOARD REVIEW

Permissions may be sought directly from Elsevier's Health Sciences Rights Department in Philadelphia, PA, USA: phone: (+1) 215 239 3804, fax: (+1) 215 239 3805, e-mail: healthpermissions@elsevier.com. You may also complete your request on-line via the Elsevier homepage (http://www.elsevier.com), by selecting 'Customer Support' and then 'Obtaining Permissions'.

Last digit is the print number: 9 8 7 6 5 4 3

Contents

Preface

When we were preparing for our board exam, we were discouraged by the lack of appropriate study manuals. The manuals available to us often contained many errors or contained questions whose style and subject matter were not on the actual exam. This motivated us to create the *Physical Therapy Board Review*, which contains 400 well-researched questions, answers, and explanations that we feel more closely follow the style of questions on the National Physical Therapy Exam (NPTE).

In preparation for the NPTE, the reader should remember that most of the questions will be "scenario" type questions. There are very few, if any, questions such as, "What nerve innervates the rectus femoris?" The question would more likely be phrased, "Which motions at the knee would be limited if there was an injury at the L2-L4 level?" Although the student must know the correct nerve and muscle combination to answer correctly, the question is presented in much more of a "real world" format, and we have followed this approach in writing the questions in this review.

Included at the front of the book is an outline of the content of the National Physical Therapy Exam. While the *Physical Therapy Board Review* does not follow this outline in all respects, we created questions from each of the major areas of the content outline. Students should use this outline to focus on weak areas of study that require further review. A bibliography of the resources used in preparing this review manual is located at the end of the book.

Brad Fortinberry, DPT, SCS
Michael Dunaway, PT

RUBRIC	CONTENT OUTLINE FOR THE NATIONAL PHYSICAL THERAPY EXAMINATION

10   **I. ASSESSMENT AND EVALUATION (24%)**

1001   **A. General Procedures (18%)**

100101   **1. Data Collection (7%)**

Obtain the following patient information and interpret implications for education:

10010101	Medical/surgical history
10010102	Special tests and diagnostic procedures (e.g., angiography, stress test, arthrogram, pulmonary function tests, roentgenogram, CT, MRI reports, sonograms, and electrocard)
10010103	Medications
10010104	Laboratory results
10010105	Psychosocial history and current status
10010106	Home environment, family and community support systems

100102   **2. Test/Measurements (11%)**

10010201	Perform selected physical therapy assessments in a safe and accurate manner including handling all monitoring devices, equipment, or lines attached to or around patient
10010202	Select and justify evaluation procedures and applications that are appropriate to the patient's status, medical diagnosis, treatment, age, functional needs, and any limiting factors
10010203	Observe the patient's response to the physical therapy assessment and treatment procedures and respond accordingly
10010204	Determine patient need for assistive devices (e.g., positional supports or mobility aids)
10010205	Perform re-evaluations based on changes in patient status as appropriate
10010206	Evaluate balance and coordination
10010207	Evaluate pain
10010208	Evaluate functional mobility
10010209	Evaluate endurance
10010210	Determine patient need for therapeutic seating or wheelchairs
10010211	Evaluate functional capacity
10010212	Evaluate cognitive function as it relates to patient's participation in PT program and attainment of goals
10010213	Perform sensory/perceptual testing
10010214	Perform structure-specific tests (e.g., vertebral impingement syndromes)
10010215	Evaluate gait
10010216	Perform manual muscle testing
10010217	Evaluate muscle performance (e.g., with equipment, isokinetics, substitution, etc.)
10010218	Identify normal and abnormal postures
10010219	Measure joint range of motion
10010220	Measure length and girth of body parts

1002	**B. System Specific Procedures (6%)**

10020001	Measure blood pressure and pulse rate during rest and exercise
10020002	Evaluate circulatory status
10020003	Evaluate status of musculoskeletal structures, soft tissue, integrity, muscle tone, joint play and flexibility
10020004	Evaluate status of skin (e.g., wounds/burns)
10020005	Evaluate pulmonary status (e.g., chest mobility, auscultation, percussion, cough, sputum
10020006	Identify heart sounds and changes
10020007	Identify patient need for orthotic or prosthetic devices
10020008	Evaluate movement patterns and motor output control
10020009	Perform electrodiagnostic testing
10020010	Evaluate neruologic status (central and peripheral and autonomic)
10020011	Evaluate achievement of developmental milestones in pediatric patients

20	**II. INTERPRETATION AND PLANNING (22%)**

2001	**A. Data Interpretation (13%)**

| 20010001 | Identify precautions and contraindications to treatment |
| 20010002 | Determine possible causes of patient's problem (i.e., relationships between patient's problems and signs and symptoms) |

2002	**B. Goal Setting and Care Planning (9%)**

20020001	Select and justify treatments and procedures
20020002	Establish measurable, short- and long-term goals, and discharge plan for patients in collaboration with patient, family, and health care team
20020003	Prioritize patient problems and associated treatments
20020004	Identify appropriate outcome measures
20020005	Identify barriers to patient progress

30	**III. INTERVENTION (54%)**

3001	**A. Preparation (10%)**

30010001	Use strategies to minimize injury to patient and therapist during treatment (such as fall, burn, injury, etc.)
30010002	Use appropriate transfer techniques and devices when transferring patients
30010003	Ensure the safety associated with the use of equipment and modalities and with the environment
30010004	Establish and/or evaluate exercise and fitness programs
30010005	Position, move, and drape patient for effective, comfortable treatment and privacy

30010006   Perform treatments to optimize responses with respect to patient's schedule for medication and other factors that could influence performance

Utilize the following
30020007   Resisted exercise with and without equipment
30020008   Passive motion/stretching exercise programs
30020009   Balance training
30020010   Fitness/conditioning/endurance exercise programs
30020011   Continuous passive motion (CPM)
30020012   Home and independent programs
30020013   Active and active assisted exercise
30020014   Aquatic exercise/therapeutic pool
30020015   Posture training
30020016   Relaxation training

Employ the following to enhance mobility and daily living activities:
30020017   Transfers with or without equipment
30020018   Gait training with or without assistive devices
30020019   Wheelchair management
30020020   Bed mobility
30020021   Adaptive devices, such as orthotics
30020022   Work simulation and retraining
30020023   Personal care activities

Apply the following:
30020024   High voltage stimulation
30020025   Interferential current
30020026   Functional electrical nerve stimulation (FES)
30020027   Low voltage stimulation
30020028   Transcutaneous electrical nerve stimulation (TENS)

Utilize the following:
30020029   Mechanical traction
30020030   Ultrasound
30020031   Hot pack
30020032   Whirlpool/Hubbard tank
30020033   Cryotherapy/cold packs/ice message
30020034   Iontophoresis
30020035   Phonophoresis
30020036   Mechanical compression/vasopneumatic devices/compression garments
30020037   Paraffin bath
30020038   Short wave diathermy
30020039   Ultraviolet
30020040   Infrared radiation
30020041   Contrast bath
30020043   Biofeedback
30020044   Apply flexible dressing/supports/elastic bandaging (e.g., for edema control, etc.)
30020045   Guide the patient in normal movement patterns
30020046   Use appropriate motivators to elicit optimal patient responses
30020047   Perform facilitation/inhibition techniques
30020048   Fabricate and adjust positioning devices
30020049   Utilize age-appropriate activities to further development

30020050	Utilize behavior modification
30020051	Apply therapeutic massage
30020052	Utilize reality orientation

Employ the following to enhance mobility and daily living activities:

30020053	Energy conservation

3003 C. Education/Communication

30030001	Educate support staff in safe and effective handling of patients and equipment related to staff duties
30030002	Educate the patient, family/significant others, and other health care personnel in safe and efficient physical therapy techniques as appropriate
30030003	Educate the patient, family/significant others, and other health care personnel about the postdischarge programs, self-management, and coping strategies
30030004	Instruct the patient clearly and concisely, including the effective use of demonstration
30030005	Explain physical therapy assessment, treatment procedures, expected outcomes and results to the patient, family/significant others and verify their understanding of same
30030006	Consult with, refer to, or educate other health care personnel in areas of physical therapy expertise
30030007	Communicate results of assessment/evaluation to physicians, the health care team, and other physical therapists
30030008	Identify patient/family education needs
30030009	Provide appropriate and timely feedback to patients, families and colleagues
30030010	Act as a resource to general public regarding health promotion, screening, and disease prevention
30030011	Document all relevant aspects of care including treatment plan, patient evaluation, and progress notes

3004 D. Supporting Activities (8%)

30040001	Respect the knowledge, rights, confidentiality, and dignity of the patient, family, and significant others
30040002	Abide by regulatory requirements and the legal and ethical standards of the profession, including quality improvement (implement established quality control standards)
30040003	Recognize the scope and limitations of self and profession
30040004	Apply principles of ethical decision making
30040005	Secure informed consent for evaluation and treatment
30040006	Procure safe and effective equipment
30040007	Delegate and supervise treatment activities as appropriate

3005 E. System-Specific Procedures (6%)

30050001	Administer oxygen

Apply the following manual therapy techniques

30050002	Joint mobilization
30050004	Soft tissue mobilization
30050005	Muscle energy

Engage in the following prosthetic (amputee) rehabilitation activities:
30050006   Residual limb bandaging
30050007   Prosthetic gait training
30050008   Care and use of prosthesis
30050009   Preprosthetic training

Utilize the following for pulmonary secretion removal:
30050010   Instillation/suctioning
30050011   Bronchial drainage techniques
30050012   Cough enhancement techniques
30050013   Mechanical devices to loosen secretions

Utilize the following to enhance respiration:
30050014   Positions to relieve dyspnea
30050015   Positions to improve ventilation/oxygenation
30050016   Breathing exercises
30050017   Respirtory muscle training with functional activities
30050018   Incentive spirometry
30050019   Perform wound cleansing and debride wounds
30050020   Apply wound coverings
30050021   Apply scar management techniques
30050022   Provide vestibular rehabilitation
30050023   Provide oral-motor stimulation
30050024   Fabricate and adjust orthoses
30050025   Utilize taping techniques

Outline reprinted with permission of the Federation of State Boards of Physical Therapy, Alexandria, Virginia

Exam Questions

Question 1.

The therapist is ambulating a patient with an above-knee amputation. The new prosthesis causes the heel on the involved foot to move laterally at toe-off. Which of the following is the most likely cause of this deviation?

A. Too much internal rotation of the prosthetic knee
B. Too much external rotation of the prosthetic knee
C. Too much outset of prosthetic foot
D. None of the above would cause this deviation

Question 2.

A therapist is testing key muscles on a patient who recently suffered a spinal cord injury. The current test assesses the strength of the long toe extensors. Which nerve segment primarily innervates this key muscle group?

A. L2
B. L3
C. L4
D. L5

Question 3.

A patient asks the therapist to explain the function of his medication verapamil (a calcium antagonist). Which of the following points should be conveyed in the therapist's explanation?

A. Verapamil causes decreased contractility of the heart and vasodilation of the coronary arteries
B. Verapamil causes decreased contractility of the heart and vasoconstriction of the coronary arteries
C. Verapamil causes increased contractility of the heart and vasodilation of the coronary arteries
D. Verapamil causes increased contractility of the heart and vasoconstriction of the coronary arteries

Question 4.

While assessing the standing posture of a patient, the therapist notes that a spinous process in the thoracic region is shifted laterally. The therapist estimates that T2 is the involved vertebra because he or she notes that it is at the approximate level of the:

A. Inferior angle of the scapula
B. Superior angle of the scapula
C. Spine of the scapula
D. Xiphoid process of the sternum

Question 5.

A patient comes to the therapist because she has noted a pronounced tuft of hair on the center of her spinal column in the lumbar area. The therapist notes no loss in motor or sensory function. This patient most likely has what form of spina bifida?

A. Meningocele
B. Meningomyelocele
C. Spina bifida occulta
D. None of the above

Question 6.

Persuading a sedentary patient to become more active, the therapist explains the benefits of exercise. Which of the following is an inappropriate list of benefits?

A. Increased efficiency of the myocardium to obtain oxygen, decreased high-density lipoprotein (HDL) cholesterol, and decreased cholesterol
B. Decreased low-density lipoprotein (LDL) cholesterol, decreased triglycerides, and decreased blood pressure
C. Increased efficiency of the myocardium to obtain oxygen, decreased cholesterol, and decreased LDL
D. Both B and C are inappropriate lists

Question 7.

A therapist is instructed to provide electrical stimulation to a patient with a venous stasis ulcer on the right lower extremity. What is the correct type of electrical stimulation to promote wound healing?

A. Biphasic pulsed current
B. Direct current
C. Interferential current
D. Transcutaneous electrical stimulation

Question 8.

While ambulating a stroke patient (the right side is the involved side), the therapist notes increased circumduction of the right lower extremity. Which of the following is an unlikely cause of this deviation?

A. Increased spasticity of the right gastrocnemius
B. Increased spasticity of the right quadriceps
C. Weak hip flexors
D. Weak knee extensors

Question 9.

Which of the following is a contraindication to ultrasound at 1.5 watts/cm^2 with a 1-MHz sound head?

A. Over a recent fracture site
B. Over noncemented metal implant
C. Over a recently surgically repaired tendon
D. Over the quadriceps muscle belly

Question 10.

The therapist is treating a 52-year-old woman after right total hip replacement. The patient complains of being self conscious about a limp. She carries a heavy briefcase to and from work every day. The therapist notes a Trendelenburg gait during ambulation on level surfaces. What advice can the therapist give the patient to minimize gait deviation?

A. Carry the briefcase in the right hand
B. Carry the briefcase in the left hand
C. The patient should not carry a briefcase at all
D. It does not matter in which hand the briefcase is carried

Question 11.

The supervisor of a rehabilitative facility insists on a weekly meeting to discuss drops in productivity. The supervisor is not concerned with the increased demand placed on the already overworked employees. According to the managerial grid, what is the best classification of this manager?

A. 5,5
B. 9,9
C. 1,9
D. 9,1

Question 12.

What is the major concern of the physical therapist treating a patient with an acute deep partial-thickness burn covering 27% of the total body? The patient was admitted to the intensive care burn unit 2 days ago.

A. Range of motion
B. Fluid retention
C. Helping the family cope with the injured patient
D. Home modifications on discharge

Question 13.

A pitcher is exercising in a clinic with a sports cord mounted behind and above his head. The pitcher simulates the pitching motion using the sports cord as resistance. Which proprioceptive neuromuscular facilitation (PNF) diagonal is the pitcher using to strengthen the muscles involved in pitching a baseball?

A. D1 extension
B. D1 flexion
C. D2 extension
D. D2 flexion

Question 14.

The therapist is evaluating a 32-year-old woman for complaints of right hip pain. The patient has injured the strongest ligament of the hip. The therapist places the patient in the prone position on the plinth and passively extends the involved hip. The therapist notes an abnormal amount of increase in passive hip extension. Which of the following ligaments is damaged?

A. Ischiofemoral ligament
B. Iliofemoral ligament (Y ligament of Bigelow)
C. Pubofemoral ligament
D. Ligamentum teres

Question 15.

While obtaining the history from a 62-year-old woman weighing 147 pounds, the therapist discovers that the patient has a history of rheumatoid arthritis. The order for outpatient physical therapy includes continuous traction due to a L2 disc protrusion. What is the best course of action for the therapist?

A. Follow the order
B. Consult with the physician because rheumatoid arthritis is a contraindication
C. Apply intermittent traction instead of continuous traction
D. Use continuous traction with the weight setting at 110 pounds

Question 16.

The therapist in an outpatient physical therapy clinic receives an order to obtain a shoe orthotic for a patient. After evaluating the patient, the therapist finds a stage I pressure ulcer on the first metatarsal head. Weight-bearing surfaces need to be transferred posteriorly. Which orthotic is the most appropriate for this patient?

A. Scaphoid pad
B. Thomas heel
C. Metatarsal pad
D. Cushion heel

Question 17.

On examination of a cross-section of the spinal cord of a cadaver, the examiner notes plaques. This finding is most characteristic of what condition?

A. Parkinson's disease
B. Myasthenia gravis
C. Multiple sclerosis
D. Dementia

Question 18.

Which of the following actions places the greatest stress on the patellofemoral joint?

A. When the foot first contacts the ground during the gait cycle
B. Exercising on a stair-stepper machine
C. Running down a smooth decline of 30°
D. Squats to 120° of knee flexion

Question 19.

A therapist working at a hospital calls another therapist in an outpatient facility to provide a brief history of a patient who is scheduled to leave the hospital and receive outpatient therapy. The acute care therapist states that the patient received an injury to the somatic sensory association cortex in one hemisphere. From this information only, the outpatient therapist knows that the patient will most likely:

A. Ignore someone talking to him or her on the involved side
B. Be unable to find one of his or her extremities
C. Have no trouble putting on clothes
D. Be unable to understand speech

Question 20.

A patient recently diagnosed with multiple sclerosis presents to a physical therapy clinic. The patient asks the therapist what she needs to avoid with this condition. Which of the following should the patient avoid?

A. Hot tubs
B. Slightly increased intake of fluids
C. Application of ice packs
D. Strength training

Question 21.

The therapist is evaluating a patient with a diagnosis of cerebral palsy. The therapist notes that all of the extremities and the trunk are involved. Further assessment also reveals that the lower extremities are more involved than the upper extremities and that the right side is more involved than the left. This patient most likely has which classification of cerebral palsy?

A. Spastic hemiplegia
B. Spastic triplegia
C. Spastic quadriplegia
D. Spastic diplegia

Question 22.

A therapist is treating a 35-year-old man diagnosed, with lumbar disc degeneration, in an outpatient clinic. Through conversation with the patient, the therapist learns that he is also being treated by a chiropractor for cervical dysfunction. What is the best course of action by the therapist?

A. Continue with the current treatment plan and ignore the chiropractor's treatment
B. Ask the patient what the chiropractor is doing and try the same approach
C. Stop physical therapy at once and consult with the referring physician
D. Contact the chiropractor to coordinate his or her plan of care with the physical therapy plan of care

Question 23.

A therapist is mobilizing a patient's right shoulder. The movement taking place at the joint capsule is not completely to end range. It is a large-amplitude movement from near the beginning of available range to near the end of available range. What grade mobilization, according to Maitland, is being performed?

A. Grade I
B. Grade II
C. Grade III
D. Grade IV

Question 24.

While observing the ambulation of a 57-year-old man with an arthritic right hip, the therapist observes a right lateral trunk lean. Why does the patient present with this gait deviation?

A. To move weight toward the involved hip and increase joint compression force
B. To move weight toward the uninvolved hip and decrease joint compression force
C. To bring the line of gravity closer to the involved hip joint
D. To take the line of gravity away from the involved hip joint

Question 25.

The therapist has given a patient an ultraviolet treatment. The patient calls the therapist the next day with complaints of peeling and itching. These signs and symptoms resolve three days later (a total of 4 days after the treatment). What dosage did the patient receive?

A. Suberythemal dose
B. Minimal erythemal dose
C. First-degree erythemal dose
D. Third-degree erythemal dose

Question 26.

Which of the following duties cannot be legally performed by a physical therapist assistant?

A. Confer with a doctor about a patient's status
B. Add 5 pounds to a patient's current exercise protocol
C. Allow a patient to increase in frequency from 2 times/week to 3 times/week
D. Perform joint mobilization

Question 27.

The therapist is treating a track athlete who specializes in sprinting and wants to increase his or her speed on the track. To accomplish this goal the plan of care should include activities to develop fast-twitch muscle fibers. Characteristics of this type fiber include:

A. Fatigues slowly, fiber colors appear red, and used more in aerobic activity
B. Fatigues quickly, fiber colors appear white, and used in anaerobic activity
C. Fatigues quickly, fiber colors appear white, and used more in aerobic activity
D. Fatigues slowly, fiber colors appear white, and used more in anaerobic activity

Question 28.

A physical therapist should place the knee in which of the following positions to palpate the lateral collateral ligament (LCL)?

A. Knee at 60° of flexion and the hip externally rotated
B. Knee at 20° of flexion and the hip at neutral
C. Knee at 90° of flexion and the hip externally rotated
D. Knee at 0° and the hip at neutral

Question 29.

The therapist receives an order to treat a 42-year-old man admitted to the hospital 3 days ago with a stab wound to the left lower thoracic spine. The patient is unable to move the left lower extremity and cannot feel pain or temperature differences in the right lower extremity. What is the most likely type of lesion?

A. Anterior cord syndrome
B. Brown-Sequard syndrome
C. Central cord syndrome
D. The patient is equally as likely to have anterior cord syndrome as he is to have Brown-Sequard syndrome

Question 30.

The therapist is working in an outpatient cardiac rehabilitation facility. A 50-year-old healthy man inquires about the correct exercise parameters for increasing aerobic efficiency. Which of the following is the most correct information to convey to this individual?

A. Exercise at 50–85% of maximal volume of oxygen utilization (VO_2)
B. Exercise with heart rate between 111 and 153 beats/minute
C. Exercise at approximately 170 beats/minute
D. A and B are correct

Question 31.

The therapist is treating a patient with a T4 spinal cord injury when the patient suddenly complains of a severe headache. The therapist also notes that the patient's pupils are constricted and that the patient is sweating profusely. Which of the following is the best course of action for the therapist?

A. Try to find a probable source of noxious stimulus and position the patient supine with feet elevated
B. Try to find a probable source of noxious stimulus and position the patient with upper trunk elevated and legs lowered
C. Try to find a probable source of noxious stimulus and place the patient in a sidelying position
D. Try to find a probable source of noxious stimulus and position the patient in prone position

Question 32.

What lobe of the lungs is the therapist attempting to drain if the patient is in the following position? Resting on the left side, rolled ¼ turn back, supported with pillows, and the foot of the bed raised 12–16 inches.

A. Right middle lobe-lingular segment
B. Left upper lobe-lingular segment
C. Right upper lobe-posterior segment
D. Left upper lobe-posterior segment

Question 33.

A therapist has been treating a patient who received a rotator cuff surgical repair with sessions consisting only of passive range of motion (for an extended period). The patient has just returned from a follow-up doctor's visit with an additional order to continue with passive range of motion only. Which of the following is the best course of action for the therapist?

A. Continue with passive range of motion as instructed, and call the physician to consult with him or her about the initiation of active range of motion
B. Begin active range of motion within the pain-free range, and continue passive range of motion
C. Continue passive range of motion, and do not question the physician's decision
D. Perform passive range of motion and any other exercise that is within the normal protocol for this diagnosis

Question 34.

A 25-year-old woman has been referred to a physical therapist by an orthopedist because of low back pain. The therapist is performing an ultrasound at the L3 level of the posterior back when the patient suddenly informs the therapist that she is looking forward to having her third child. On further investigation, the therapist discovers that the patient is in the first trimester of pregnancy. Which of the following is the best course of action for the therapist?

A. Change the settings of the ultrasound from continuous to pulsed
B. Continue with the continuous setting because first-trimester pregnancy is not a contraindication
C. Cease treatment, notify the patient's orthopedic physician, and document the mistake
D. Send the patient to the gynecologist for an immediate sonogram

Question 35.

A 29-year-old woman is referred to a therapist with a diagnosis of recurrent ankle sprains. The patient has a history of several inversion ankle sprains within the past year. No edema or redness is noted at this time. Which of the following is the best treatment plan?

A. Gastrocnemius stretching, ankle strengthening, and ice
B. Rest, ice, compression, elevation, and ankle strengthening
C. Ankle strengthening and a proprioception program
D. Rest, ice, compression, elevation, and gastrocnemius stretching

Question 36.

The therapist is treating a patient in an outpatient facility for strengthening of bilateral lower extremities. During the initial assessment the patient reveals that he has a form of cancer but is reluctant to offer any other information about his medical history. After 1 week of treatment, the therapist is informed by the physician that the patient has Kaposi's sarcoma and AIDS. Which of the following is the best course of action for the therapist?

A. Cease treatment of the patient, and inform him that an outpatient facility is not the appropriate environment for a person with his particular medical condition
B. Continue treatment of the patient in the gym, avoiding close contact with other patients and taking appropriate universal precautions
C. Continue treatment of the patient in the gym as before, taking appropriate universal precautions
D. Cease treatment, but do not confront the patient with the knowledge of his HIV status

Question 37.

A patient reports to therapy stating that his "sugar is too high" for exercise. What is the minimal blood glucose level that is considered too high for a diabetic patient to begin exercise?

A. 300 mg/dl
B. 400 µg/dl
C. 300 µg/dl
D. 400 mg/dl

Question 38.

The therapist is ordered to evaluate a patient in the intensive care unit. The patient appears to be in a coma and is totally unresponsive to noxious, visual, and auditory stimuli. What rating on the Rancho Los Amigos Cognitive Functioning Scale is most appropriate?

A. I
B. III
C. IV
D. VIV

Question 39.

A patient presents to an outpatient physical therapy clinic with a severed ulnar nerve of the right upper extremity. What muscle is still active and largely responsible for the obvious hyperextension at the metacarpophalangeal (MCP) joints of the involved hand?

A. Dorsal interossei
B. Volar interossei
C. Extensor carpi radialis brevis
D. Extensor digitorum

Question 40.

A physician notes a vertebral fracture in the x-ray of a patient involved in a car accident. The fractured vertebra has a bifid spinous process. Which of the following vertebrae is the most likely to be involved?

A. Fourth lumbar vertebra
B. Fifth cervical vertebra
C. Twelfth thoracic vertebra
D. First sacral vertebra

Question 41.

The therapist routinely places ice on the ankle of a patient with an acute ankle sprain. Ice application has many therapeutic benefits. Which of the following is the body's first response to application of ice?

A. Vasoconstriction of local vessels
B. Decreased nerve condition velocity
C. Decreased local sensitivity
D. All occur simultaneously

Question 42.

The therapist is evaluating a patient with left-side visual field deficits in both eyes. A lesion at what location may cause this deficit?

A. At the optic chiasm
B. At the right side optic tract
C. At the left side optic nerve
D. At the right side optic nerve

Question 43.

According to the Joint Commission on Accreditation of Health Care Organizations (JCAHO), what is a sentinel event?

A. A patient who is seriously injured at a facility
B. An employee who is seriously injured at a facility
C. A JCAHO surveyor who finds a major error in a facility's billing policies
D. A JCAHO surveyor who finds a major error in the structure of a facility (e.g., not enough handicap parking, not enough wheel chair ramps)

Question 44.

A patient presents to an outpatient facility with complaints of pain in the groin area (along the medial left thigh). With manual muscle testing of the involved lower extremity a therapist determines the following: hip flexion = 4+/5, hip extension = 4+/5, hip abduction = 4+/5, hip adduction = 2+/5, hip internal rotation = 2+/5, and hip external rotation = 2+/5. Which nerve on the involved side is most likely injured?

A. Lateral cutaneous nerve of the upper thigh
B. Obturator nerve
C. Femoral nerve
D. Ilioinguinal nerve

Question 45.

The therapist is treating a male patient for a second-degree acromioclavicular sprain. The patient has just finished the doctor's prescription of 3 sessions/week for 4 weeks. The therapist is treating the patient with iontophoresis (driving dexamethasone), deltoid-strengthening exercises, pectoral-strengthening exercises, and ice. The patient reports no decline in pain level since the initial evaluation. Which of the following is the best course of action for the therapist?

A. Phone the doctor and request continued physical therapy
B. Tell the patient to go back to the doctor because he is not making appropriate progress
C. Discharge the patient because he will improve on his own
D. Take the problem to the supervisor of the facility

Question 46.

The protocol for a cardiac patient states that the patient should not exceed 5 metabolic equivalents (METs) with any activity at this stage of recovery. Which of the following activities would be inappropriate for the patient?

A. Cycling 11 miles per hour
B. Walking 4 miles per hour
C. Driving a car
D. Weeding a garden

Question 47.

Which of the following is a correct statement about Medicare?

A. Medicare Part A is only for patients over 85 years old
B. Medicare Part B is only for patients 65–84 years old
C. Medicare Part A is only for inpatient treatment
D. Medicare Part B is only for use in long-term facilities

Question 48.

A mother comes to a therapist concerned that her 4-month-old infant cannot sit up alone yet. Which of the following responses is the most appropriate for the therapist?

A. "Your infant probably needs further evaluation by a specialist because, although it varies, infants can usually sit unsupported at 2 months of age"
B. "Your infant probably needs further evaluation by a specialist because, although it varies, infants can usually sit unsupported at 3 months of age"
C. "This is probably nothing to be concerned about because, although it varies, most infants can sit unsupported at 8 months of age"
D. "This is probably nothing to be concerned about because, although it varies, most infants can sit unsupported at 5 months at age"

Question 49.

A therapist decides to buy two ultrasound machines from a sales representative. The representative offers the therapist a free steak dinner at a local restaurant as a token of appreciation. What is the best course of action for the therapist?

A. Refuse the dinner gracefully
B. Take his or her family out to eat
C. Offer to take the representative out to dinner
D. Take a local doctor out to dinner and discuss the benefits of using this type of ultrasound

Question 50.

While observing a patient with posttraumatic brain injury (TBI), the therapist notes an increase in left ankle plantar flexion during loading response (heel strike to foot flat) of the involved lower extremity. With this particular patient, the left side is the involved side. Which of the following is not a likely cause of this deviation?

A. Spasticity of the left gastrocnemius
B. Hypotonicity of the left tibialis anterior
C. Leg length discrepancy
D. Left quadricep hypertonicity

Question 51.

A therapist working in an outpatient physical therapy clinic evaluates a patient with a diagnosis of rotator cuff bursitis. The physician's order is to evaluate and treat. During the evaluation the following facts are revealed:

• Active shoulder flexion = 85° with pain
• Passive shoulder flexion = 177°
• Active shoulder abduction = 93° with pain
• Passive shoulder abduction = 181°
• Active external rotation = 13° with pain
• Passive eternal rotation = 87°
• Drop arm test = positive
• Impingement test = negative
• Biceps tendon subluxation test = negative
• Sulcus sign = negative

Of the following, which is the best course of action?

A. Treat the patient for 1 week with moist heat application, joint mobilization, and strengthening. Then suggest to the patient that he or she return to the physician if there are no positive results.
B. Treat the patient for 1 week with ultrasound, strengthening, and ice. Then suggest to the patient that he or she return to the physician if there are no positive results.
C. Treat the patient for 1 week with a home exercise program, strengthening, passive range of motion by the therapist, and ice. Then suggest to the patient that he or she return to the physician if there are no positive results.
D. Treat the patient for 1 week with strengthening, a home exercise program, and ice. Then suggest to the patient that he or she return to the physician if there are no positive results.

Question 52.

A patient's lawyer calls the therapist requesting his or her client's clinical records. The lawyer states that he or she needs the records to pay the patient's bill. What is the best course of action?

A. Tell the lawyer either to have the patient request a copy of the records or to have the patient sign a medical release.
B. Fax the needed chart to the lawyer.
C. Mail a copy of the chart to the patient.
D. Call the patient and tell him or her of the recent development.

Question 53.

A local plant asks a therapy team to perform a study of its workers. The study needs to determine the frequency of lung cancer in workers who insulate the inside area of an electrical oven appliance. Using company files, the therapy team studies all past employees with this job description. The employees were initially free of lung cancer, as determined by a routine physician's examination required by the plant. The team records from these files the frequency with which each one of the employees developed lung cancer. What type of study is the therapy team performing?

A. Historical prospective
B. Historical cohort
C. Case control
D. A & B

Question 54.

CORF is an abbreviation for which of the following?

A. Certified Owner of a Rehabilitation Facility.
B. Certified Outpatient Rehabilitation Facility.
C. Control Organization for Rehabilitation Facilities.
D. Corporation for Organization of Rehabilitation Facilities.

Question 55.

The therapist is crutch-training a 26-year-old man who underwent right knee arthroscopy 10 hours ago. The patient's weight-bearing status is toe-touch weight-bearing on the right lower extremity. If the patient is going up steps, which of the following is the correct sequence of verbal instructions?

A. "Have someone stand below you while going up, bring the left leg up first, then the crutches and the right leg"
B. "Have someone stand above you while going up, bring the left leg up first, then the crutches and the right leg"
C. "Have someone stand below you while going up, bring the right leg up first, then the crutches and the left leg"
D. "Have someone stand above you while going up, bring the right leg up first, then the crutches and the right leg"

Question 56.

A 35-year-old woman with a diagnosis of lumbar strain has a physician's prescription with a frequency and duration of 3 sessions/week for 6 weeks. The physical therapy evaluation reveals radiculopathy into the L5 dermatome of the right lower extremity, increased radiculopathy with lumbar flexion, decreased radiculopathy with lumbar extension, poor posture, and hamstring tightness bilaterally at 60°. What is the best course of treatment?

A. Lumbar traction, hot packs, and ultrasound.
B. McKenzie style lumbar extensions, a posture program, hamstring stretching, and a home exercise program.
C. McKenzie style lumbar extensions, a posture program, hamstring stretching, home program, hot packs, and ultrasound.
D. Lumbar traction, hot packs, ultrasound, and hamstring stretching.

Question 57.

A therapist is examining a 3-year-old child, who is positioned as follows: supine, hips flexed to 90°, hips fully adducted, and knees flexed. The therapist passively abducts and raises the thigh, applying an anterior shear force to the hip joint. A click at 30° of abduction is noted by the therapist. What orthopedic test is the therapist performing, and what is its significance?

A. Ortolani's test—hip dislocation
B. Appley's compression/distraction test—cartilage damage
C. McMurray test—cartilage damage
D. Piston test—hip dislocation

Question 58.

A teenager comes to an outpatient facility with complaints of pain at the tibial tubercle when playing basketball. The therapist notices that the tubercles are abnormally pronounced on bilateral knees. What condition does the patient most likely have?

A. Jumper's knees
B. Anterior cruciate ligament sprain
C. Osgood-Schlatter disease
D. A & C

Question 59.

What is the best way to first exercise the postural (or extensor) musculature when it is extremely weak to facilitate muscle control?

A. Isometrically
B. Concentrically
C. Eccentrically
D. Isokinetically

Question 60.

A patient presents to physical therapy with complaints of pain in the right hip due to osteoarthritis. Which of the following is not true about this type of arthritis?

A. Causes pain usually symmetrically because it is a systemic condition
B. Not usually more painful in the morning
C. This type of arthritis commonly involves the distal interphalangeal joint
D. Mainly involves weight-bearing joints

Question 61.

Which of the following is observed by the therapist if a patient is correctly performing an anterior pelvic tilt in standing position?

A. Hip extension and lumbar flexion
B. Hip flexion and lumbar extension
C. Hip flexion and lumbar flexion
D. Hip extension and lumbar extension

Question 62.

Which of the following is used to treat a patient referred to physical therapy with a diagnosis of Dupuytren's contracture?

A. Knee continuous passive motion (CPM)
B. Work simulator set for squatting activities
C. Hand splint
D. A two-pound dumbbell

Question 63.

If the line of gravity is posterior to the hip joint in standing, on what does the body first rely to keep the trunk from moving into excessive lumbar extension?

A. Iliopsoas muscle activity
B. Abdominal muscle activity
C. Anterior pelvic ligaments and the hip joint capsule
D. Posterior pelvic ligaments and the hip joint capsule

Question 64.

The therapist receives a referral to evaluate a patient with a boutonnière deformity. With this injury the involved finger usually presents in the position of:

A. Flexion of the proximal interphalangeal (PIP) joint and flexion of the distal interphalangeal (DIP) joint.
B. Extension of the PIP joint and flexion of the DIP joint.
C. Flexion of the PIP joint and extension of the DIP joint.
D. Extension of the PIP joint and extension of the DIP joint.

Question 65.

Which of the following is the most important to assess first during an evaluation of a patient with a recent stroke?

A. Sensory status
B. Motor control
C. Mental status
D. Ambulation potential

Question 66.

A therapist receives an order to evaluate a 72-year-old woman who has suffered a recent stroke. The therapist needs to focus on pregait activities. Which of the proprioceptive neuromuscular facilitation (PNF) diagonals best encourages normal gait?

A. D1
B. D2
C. PNF is contraindicated
D. Pelvic PNF patterns only

Question 67.

A therapist receives an order to evaluate and treat a 76-year-old woman who was involved in a motor vehicle accident 2 days ago. The patient's vehicle was struck in the rear by another vehicle. The patient has normal sensation and strength in bilateral lower extremities but paralysis and loss of sensation in bilateral upper extremities. Bowel and bladder function are normal. The patient most likely has what type of spinal cord injury?

A. Anterior cord syndrome
B. Brown-Sequard syndrome
C. Central cord syndrome
D. There is no evidence of an incomplete spinal cord lesion

Question 68.

A patient living in a nursing home with Medicare part A as the source of reimbursement is treated by physical therapy only. What is the required minimal frequency of physical therapy treatment?

A. One time/week
B. Three times/week
C. Five times/week
D. There is no required time frame

Question 69.

At what point in the gait cycle is the center of gravity the lowest?

A. Double support
B. Terminal swing
C. Deceleration
D. Mid-stance

Question 70.

A twelve year old male has been referred to physical therapy after recently being involved in a car accident. The patient's mother has signed all the necessary paperwork for admission to the clinic, including a form allowing release of her son's records to the parties listed. The patient's mother included herself, doctors involved in the patient's care, and their attorney on the list. The patient's stepfather comes to the clinic after the patient is discharged and requests a copy of the stepson's record. Which of the following would be the correct response from the office staff?

A. Give the stepfather a copy of the records.
B. Give the stepfather a copy of the records after he has signed a release form.
C. Inform the patient's stepfather that he is not on the list that authorizes the records to be released to him.
D. Call the patient's mother and get verbal permission to release the records to the stepfather.

Question 71.

A therapist is working in an outpatient rehabilitation facility. A female patient presents with an order for occupational therapy to evaluate and treat a diagnosis of carpal tunnel syndrome. The occupational therapist (OT) brings to the attention of the physical therapist (PT) that the patient's insurance will not reimburse for occupational therapy services. What is the best course of action?

A. Allow the OT to treat the patient and the PT to sign off on his or her work.
B. Tell the patient that she will have to pay out of pocket for OT services.
C. Call the doctor's office and obtain an order for PT, then allow the PT to treat the patient.
D. Tell the patient to return to her doctor to obtain a PT order.

Question 72.

The home health physical therapist arrives late at the home of a patient for a treatment session just as the occupational therapist has finished. The patient is angry because the sessions are so close together. The patient becomes verbally abusive toward the physical therapist. The most appropriate response to the patient is:

A. "I'm sorry I'm late, but you must try to understand that I am extremely busy."
B. "I know you are aggravated. It is inconvenient when someone does not show up when expected. Let's just do our best this session and I will make an effort to see that we do not have PT and OT scheduled so close together from now on."
C. "You have to expect visits at any time of the day with home health."
D. "The OT and I did not purposefully arrive so close together. I apologize, please let's now begin therapy."

Question 73.

Which of the following is not an acceptable long-term goal for a patient with a complete C7 spinal cord injury?

A. Independence with dressing
B. Driving an automobile
C. Balance a wheelchair for 30 seconds using a "wheelie"
D. Independence with performing a manual cough

Question 74.

A 17-year-old football player is referred to the outpatient physical therapy clinic with a diagnosis of a recent third-degree medial collateral ligament sprain of the knee. The patient wishes to return to playing football as soon as possible. Which of the below is the best protocol?

A. Fit the patient with a brace that prevents him from actively moving the knee into the last available 20° of extension. Prescribe general lower extremity strengthening with the exception of sidelying hip adduction.
B. Do not fit the patient with a brace. All lower extremity strengthening exercises are indicated.
C. Fit the patient with a brace that prevents him from actively moving the knee into the last available 20° of extension. Avoid all open-chain strengthening for the lower extremity.
D. Do not fit the patient with a brace. Prescribe general lower extremity strengthening with the exception of sidelying hip adduction.

Question 75.

The therapist is working in a nursing home. The company for which the therapist works requires that therapists be at least 75% efficient. The therapist realizes that he or she cannot effectively treat the patients in the given time frame. What is the best course of action?

A. Work until the 75% limit is up and cease treatment
B. Work with the patients until the 75% limit is up and complete paperwork for the rest of the 8 hour working day
C. Quit the job and find a company that does not require the 75% limit
D. Go to the immediate supervisor in an attempt to alleviate the problem

Question 76.

In an attempt to establish a home exercise program the therapist gives a patient written exercises. After 1 week, the patient returns and has not performed any of the exercises. After further questioning, the therapist determines that the patient is illiterate. What is the best course of action?

A. Go over the exercises in a one-on-one review session
B. Give the patient a picture of the exercises
C. Give a copy of the exercises to a literate family member
D. All of the above

Question 77.

How often does the Joint Commission on Accreditation of Healthcare Organizations (JCAHO) survey hospitals?

A. Once per year
B. Every 2 years
C. Every 3 years
D. Every 5 years

Question 78.

What is the closed-packed position of the shoulder?

A. Internal rotation and abduction
B. External rotation and abduction
C. Internal rotation and adduction
D. External rotation and adduction

Question 79.

A 42-year-old receptionist presents to an outpatient physical therapy clinic complaining of low back pain. The therapist decides that postural modification needs to be part of the treatment plan. What is the best position for the lower extremities while the patient is sitting?

A. 90° of hip flexion, 90° of knee flexion, and 10° of dorsiflexion
B. 60° of hip flexion, 90° of knee flexion, and 0° of dorsiflexion
C. 110° of hip flexion, 80° of knee flexion, and 10° of dorsiflexion
D. 90° of hip flexion, 90° of knee flexion, and 0° of dorsiflexion

Question 80.

The therapist works in a cardiac rehabilitation setting. Which of the following types of exercises are most likely to be harmful to a 64-year-old man with a history of myocardial infarction?

A. Concentric
B. Eccentric
C. Aerobic
D. Isometric

Question 81.

A 50-year-old man has a persistent cough, purulent sputum, abnormal dilation of bronchi, more frequent involvement of the left lower lobe than the right, hemoptysis, and reduced forced vital capacity. What is the most likely pulmonary dysfunction?

A. Chronic bronchitis
B. Emphysema
C. Asthma
D. Bronchiectasis

Question 82.

The following is a long-term goal for a patient with spinal cord injury: independence in performing a manual cough without applying pressure to the abdomen. This goal is the most challenging and obtainable for a patient with a complete lesion at which of the following spinal cord levels?

A. C5
B. C7
C. T2
D. T10

Question 83.

When ordering a customized wheelchair for a patient, the therapist determines that the pelvic belt needs to be positioned so that it allows active anterior pelvic tilt. What is the best position for the pelvic belt in relation to the sitting surface?

A. 30°
B. 45°
C. 60°
D. 90°

Question 84.

When should a physical therapist begin discharge planning for a patient admitted to a rehabilitation unit with a diagnosis of a recent stroke?

A. At the first team meeting
B. At the last team meeting
C. Two weeks before discharge
D. After the initial evaluation by the physical therapist

Question 85.

Which of the following neural fibers are the largest and fastest?

A. C fibers
B. A fibers
C. A and C are equal
D. None of the above

Question 86.

A patient with a diagnosis of a rotator cuff tear has just begun active range of motion. The therapist is strengthening the rotator cuff muscles to increase joint stability and oppose the superior shear of the deltoid. Which of the rotator cuff muscles participate least in a opposing the superior shear force of the deltoid?

A. Infraspinatus
B. Subscapularis
C. Teres minor
D. Supraspinatus

Question 87.

Which of the following is an example of a policy in a physical therapy clinic?

A. No shorts worn in the clinic
B. The correct way to accept a telephone referral
C. The clinic will open at 8:00 AM
D. A and C

Question 88.

What portion of the adult knee meniscus is vascularized?

A. Outer edges
B. Inner edges
C. The entire meniscus is vascular
D. The entire meniscus is avascular

Question 89.

A 14-year-old girl with right thoracic scoliosis is referred to physical therapy. The therapist should expect which of the following findings?

A. Left shoulder high, left scapula prominent, and right hip high
B. Left shoulder low, right scapula prominent, and left hip high
C. Right shoulder high, right scapula prominent, and right hip high
D. Right shoulder low, right scapula prominent, and left hip high

Question 90.

What is the most likely cause of anterior pelvic tilt during initial contact (heel strike)?

A. Weak abdominals
B. Tight hamstrings.
C. Weak abductors
D. Back pain

Question 91.

To treat effectively most patients with Parkinson's disease, the therapist should emphasize which proprioceptive neuromuscular facilitation (PNF) pattern for the upper extremities?

A. D2 extension
B. D2 flexion
C. D1 extension
D. D1 flexion

Question 92.

Which of the following are tests for peripheral arterial involvement in a patient with complaints of calf musculature pain?

A. Claudication time
B. Homan's sign
C. Percussion test
D. None of the above

Question 93.

The therapist is asked to evaluate a baseball pitcher's rotator cuff isokinetically. Which isokinetic evaluation is most appropriate?

A. 190°/second, 180°/second, and 240°/second.
B. 30°/second, 60°/second, and 90°/second.
C. 60°/second, 120°/second, and 180°/second.
D. 180°/second, 240°/second, and 360°/second.

Question 94.

A patient presents to a clinic with decreased tidal volume (TV). What is the most likely cause of this change in normal pulmonary function?

A. Chronic obstructive pulmonary disease
B. Restrictive lung dysfunction
C. Both of the above
D. None of the above

Question 95.

The patient is referred by a physician to begin outpatient cardiac rehabilitation. Which of the following is not a contraindication to enter an outpatient program?

A. Resting systolic blood pressure of 210 mmHg
B. Third-degree atrioventricular block
C. Resting ST displacement less than 1 mm
D. Acute fever

Question 96.

In order to determine if an exercise session should be terminated, the patient is asked to assess level of exertion using the Borg Rating of Perceived Exertion Scale (RPE). The patient rates the level of exertion as 9 on the 6–19 scale. A rating of 9 corresponds to which of the following?

A. Very, very light
B. Very light
C. Somewhat hard
D. Hard

Question 97.

The therapist is treating a patient who has suffered a recent stroke. There is a significant lack of dorsiflexion in the involved lower extremity and a significant amount of medial/lateral ankle instability. The therapist believes that an ankle foot orthosis (AFO) would be beneficial. Which of the following is an appropriate AFO?

A. Solid AFO
B. Posterior leaf spring AFO
C. Hinged solid AFO
D. A or C

Question 98.

The therapist is treating a new patient with a diagnosis of lateral epicondylitis. The therapist decides to use iontophoresis driving dexamethasone. Dexamethasone is an _____ and is administered with the _____.

A. Analgesic, anode
B. Analgesic, cathode
C. Anti-inflammatory, anode
D. Anti-inflammatory, cathode

Question 99.

At what age does a human have the greatest amount of fluid in the intervertebral disc?

A. 1 year
B. 4 years
C. 7 years
D. 10 years

Question 100.

During the opening of a patient's mouth, a palpable and audible click is discovered in the left temporomandibular joint. The physician informs the therapist that the patient has an anteriorly dislocated disk. This click most likely signifies:

A. The condyle is sliding anterior to obtain normal relationship with the disk
B. The condyle is sliding posterior to obtain normal relationship with the disk
C. The condyle is sliding anterior and losing normal relationship with the disk
D. The condyle is sliding posterior and losing normal relationship with the disk

Question 101.

In what position should the therapist place the upper extremity to palpate the supraspinatus tendon?

A. Full abduction, full flexion, and full external rotation
B. Full abduction, full flexion, and full internal rotation
C. Full adduction, full external rotation, and full extension
D. Full adduction, full internal rotation, and full extension

Question 102.

What ligament is most involved in sustaining the longitudinal arch of the foot?

A. Plantar calcaneonavicular ligament
B. Long plantar ligament
C. Plantar calcaneocuboid ligament
D. Anterior talofibular ligament

Question 103.

A posterior lateral herniation of the lumbar disc between vertebrae L4 and L5 most likely results in damage to which nerve root?

A. L4
B. L5
C. L4 and L5
D. L5 and S1

Question 104.

During evaluation of a patient, the therapist observes significant posterior trunk lean at initial contact (heel strike). Which of the following is the most likely muscle that the therapist needs to focus on during the exercise session in order to minimize this gait deviation?

A. Gluteus medius
B. Gluteus maximus
C. Quadriceps
D. Hamstrings

Question 105.

A 31-year-old man has loss of vision in one eye, staggering gait, numbness in bilateral upper extremities, and decreased bowel and bladder control. The episodes of the above symptoms have occurred every few weeks for the past 6 months. Each episode has been slightly worse than the last. What is the most likely condition?

A. Parkinson's disease
B. Guillain-Barré syndrome
C. Multiple sclerosis
D. Amyotrophic lateral sclerosis

Question 106.

The use of compression stockings on the feet and ankles is contraindicated in which patient population?

A. Chronic venous disease
B. Recent total knee replacement
C. Burn patients
D. Chronic arterial disease

Question 107.

Which of the following is the best and first treatment for a wound with black eschar over 90% of the wound bed?

A. Lidocaine
B. Dexamethasone
C. Silvadene
D. Elase

Question 108.

To decrease the risk of hypoglycemia in a patient with type I insulin-dependent diabetes, which of the following is inappropriate?

A. Eat or drink a snack high in carbohydrates 30 minutes before exercise
B. Exercise muscles that have not had an insulin injection recently
C. A carbohydrate snack for each 30–45 minutes of exercise
D. Exercise at the peak time of insulin effect

Question 109.

A patient presents to an outpatient physical therapy clinic with a 140° kyphoscoliotic curve. What is the therapist's greatest concern?

A. The patient's complaint of low back pain
B. Gait deviations
C. Pulmonary status
D. Poor upright standing posture

Question 110.

A patient presents with tachypnea, corpulmonale, hypoxemia, rales on inspiration, and decreased diffusing capacity. What is the probable cause?

A. Restrictive lung dysfunction
B. Chronic obstructive pulmonary disease
C. Neither of the above
D. A and B

Question 111.

A therapist is evaluating a patient in the intensive care unit. The therapist notes no eye opening, no verbal response, and no motor response. On the Glasgow coma scale, what is the patient's score?

A. 0
B. 3
C. 5
D. 9

Question 112.

A 68-year-old man, who suffered a stroke 4 weeks ago (involving the dominant hemisphere) presents with contralateral hemiparesis and sensory loss (greater in the lower extremity than the upper extremity), mental confusion, and aphasia. What is the most likely location of the infarction?

A. Middle cerebral artery
B. Internal carotid artery
C. Posterior cerebral artery
D. Anterior cerebral artery

Question 113.

A therapist is treating an acute full-thickness burn on the entire right lower extremity of a 27-year-old man. What movements need to be stressed with splinting, positioning, and exercise to avoid contractures?

A. Hip flexion, knee extension, and ankle dorsiflexion
B. Hip extension, knee flexion, and ankle plantarflexion
C. Hip extension, knee extension, and ankle dorsiflexion
D. Hip flexion, knee extension, and ankle plantarflexion

Question 114.

A local orthopedic doctor, who is a main referral source for an outpatient clinic, insists on an all open-chain exercise program for all patients who have undergone anterior cruciate ligament reconstruction. The therapist feels a closed- and open-chain program is the best course of therapy. What is the best course of action to convince the doctor?

A. Call the physician's nurse and discuss with him or her the new treatment protocol
B. Schedule a face-to-face meeting with the doctor to discuss the correct treatmen plan
C. Fax the doctor research supporting use of a combined open- and closed-chain program
D. Have one of the doctor's colleagues convince him that the new protocol is best

Question 115.

The therapist's nephew, who is a prospect for a local minor league baseball team, wants an opinion about a set of exercises that he was given by a friend. What is the best way for the therapist to approach this situation?

A. The therapist should tell the nephew to make an appointment at the outpatient clinic
B. The therapist should have the nephew fax the exercises to the clinic; then the therapist should mark through the incorrect ones
C. The therapist should have the nephew contact his doctor for an opinion
D. The therapist should meet with the nephew after hours and discuss the exercises

Question 116.

A supervisor in a physical therapy clinic observes a new graduate performing incorrect exercises on a patient. The exercises are not life-threatening but are incorrect. What is the best way to handle this situation?

A. The supervisor should immediately tell the new therapist to stop exercising the patient and instruct the patient and therapist in the correct procedure
B. The supervisor should tactfully tell the new therapist to come into his or her office and discuss the situation in private
C. The supervisor should put a note on the new therapist's desk to meet with him/her after work
D. The supervisor should give the new therapist research articles about the correct options

Question 117.

Which of the following is the most energy-efficient and allows a T1 complete paraplegic the most functional mobility during locomotion?

A. Manual wheelchair
B. Electric wheelchair
C. Bilateral knee-ankle orthoses and crutches
D. Bilateral ankle-foot orthoses and crutches

Question 118.

Which of the following theories support the use of a transcutaneous electrical nerve stimulation (TENS) unit for sensory level pain control?

A. Gate control theory
B. Sensory interaction theory
C. Central summation theory
D. None of the above

Question 119.

After performing an evaluation, a therapist notes the following information: severe spasticity of plantar flexors in the involved lower extremity; complete loss of active dorsiflexion in the involved lower extremity; minimal spasticity between 0° and 5° of dorsiflexion, with increased spasticity when the ankle is taken into more than 5° of dorsiflexion. Which ankle-foot orthosis (AFO) is most likely contraindicated for the patient, an 87-year-old man who had a stroke 4 weeks ago?

A. Dorsiflexion spring assist AFO
B. Posterior leaf spring AFO
C. Hinged AFO
D. Spiral AFO

Question 120.

Which of the following is not an example of a synarthrodial joint in the body?

A. Coronal suture
B. The fibrous joint between the shaft of the tibia and fibula
C. Symphysis pubis
D. Metacarpophalangeal.

Question 121.

In the geriatric population, _____ *usually* occurs after _____ is present.

A. Spondylolisthesis, spondylolysis
B. Spondylolysis, spondylolisthesis
C. Spondyloschisis, spondylolysis
D. Spondylolisthesis, spondyloschisis

Question 122.

A 67-year-old woman presents to an outpatient facility with a diagnosis of right adhesive capsulitis. The therapist plans to focus mostly on gaining abduction range of motion. In which direction should the therapist mobilize the shoulder to gain abduction range of motion?

A. Posteriorly
B. Anteriorly
C. Inferiorly
D. Superiorly

Question 123.

A 13-year-old girl has fractured the left patella during a volleyball game. The physician determines that the superior pole is the location of the fracture. Which of the following should be avoided in early rehabilitation?

A. Full knee extension
B. 45° of knee flexion
C. 90° of knee flexion
D. 15° of knee flexion

Question 124.

The most common type of stroke is _____, and its primary precipitating factor is _____.

A. Atherothrombotic, atherosclerosis
B. Atherothrombotic, hypertension
C. Hemorrhagic, atherosclerosis.
D. Hemorrhagic, hypertension

Question 125.

A football player presents to an outpatient clinic with complaints of pain in the right knee after an injury suffered the night before. The physician determines that the anterior cruciate ligament (ACL) is torn. Which of the following is most commonly associated with an injury causing damage to the ACL only?

A. Varus blow to the knee with the foot planted and an audible pop
B. Foot planted, medial tibial rotation, and an audible pop
C. Valgus blow to the knee with the foot planted and no audible pop
D. Foot planted, lateral tibial rotation, and no audible pop

Question 126.

A patient is referred to the therapist with a diagnosis of arthritis. What type of arthritis would the therapist expect if the patient presented with the following signs and symptoms? (1) Bilateral wrists and knees are involved, (2) pain at rest and with motion, (3) prolonged morning stiffness, and (4) crepitus.

A. Osteoarthritis
B. Rheumatoid arthritis
C. Degenerative joint disease
D. It is not possible to determine with the given information

Question 127.

A patient presents to an outpatient clinic with complaints of shoulder pain. The therapist observes a painful arc between 70° and 120° of active abduction in the involved shoulder. This finding is most indicative of what shoulder pathology?

A. Rotator cuff tear
B. Acromioclacivular joint separation
C. Impingement
D. Labrum tear

Question 128.

A 35-year-old woman suffered brain injury in a motor vehicle accident and presents with the following symptoms: an intention tremor, nystagmus, hypotonia, and dysdiadochokinesia. What is the most likely location of the lesion?

A. Basal ganglia
B. Dorsal columns
C. Frontal lobe
D. Cerebellum

Question 129.

A tennis player receives a surgical repair of the annular ligament. Where should the therapist expect to note the most edema?

A. Radial ulnar joint
B. Olecranon bursa
C. Ulnohumeral joint
D. Lateral triangle

Question 130.

A therapist is teaching a family how to care for a family member at home. The patient is totally bed-bound. To prevent pressure ulcers most effectively, what should be the maximal amount of time between position changes?

A. One hour
B. Two hours
C. Six hours
D. Eight hours

Question 131.

While reviewing a chart before performing postural drainage and percussion, the therapist finds that the patient has a platelet count of approximately 45,000. What is the appropriate course of action?

A. Proceed with treatment
B. Call the doctor and discuss the treatment plan
C. Immediately discharge the patient from physical therapy
D. Inform nursing of the relative contraindication and proceed with treatment

Question 132.

A physician orders stage II cardiac rehabilitation for a patient. The orders are to exercise the patient below 7 metabolic equivalents (METs). Which of the following is a contraindicated activity?

A. Riding a stationary bike at approximately 5.5 mph
B. Descending a flight of stairs independently
C. Ironing
D. Ambulate independently at 5–6 mph

Question 133.

The therapist is evaluating a 36-year-old woman to fit her with the appropriate wheelchair. Recent injury caused C6 quadriplegia. What is the correct way to measure length of the footrests for the patient's permanent wheelchair?

A. From the patient's popliteal fossa to the heel and add 1 inch
B. From the patient's popliteal fossa to the heel and subtract 1 inch
C. From the patient's popliteal fossa to the first metatarsal head and add 1 inch
D. From the patient's popliteal fossa to the first metatarsal head and subtract 1 inch

Question 134.

Which of the following is least likely in a woman in the eighth month of pregnancy?

A. Center of gravity anteriorly displaced
B. Heart rate decreased with rest and increased with activity (compared to heart rate prior to pregnancy)
C. Edema in bilateral lower extremities
D. Blood pressure increased by 5% (compared with blood pressure before pregnancy)

Question 135.

In developing the plan of care for a 28-year-old pregnant woman which of the following muscles should be the focus of the strengthening exercises to maintain a strong pelvic floor?

A. Piriformis, obturator internus, and pubococcygeus
B. Obturator internus, pubococcygeus, and coccygeus
C. Rectus abdominis, iliococcygeus, and piriformis
D. Iliococcygeus, pubococcygeus, and coccygeus

Question 136.

The therapist has just returned from an inservice offering new treatment techniques in wound care. The therapist would like to share the information with interested members of the hospital staff. What is the best way to share this information?

A. Prepare a handout on the new treatment techniques and give it to the members of the hospital staff
B. Schedule a mandatory inservice during lunch for the entire hospital staff that participate in some form of wound care
C. Post bulletins in view of all hospital staff and send memos to the department heads inviting everyone to attend an inservice during lunch
D. Call each department head and invite him or her and their staff to an inservice during lunch

Question 137.

A 42-year-old construction worker received a burst fracture in the cervical spine when struck by a falling cross-beam. Proprioception is intact in bilateral lower extremities. The patient has bilateral loss of motor function and sensitivity to pain and temperature below the level of the lesion. This type of lesion is most typical of which of the following syndromes?

A. Central cord syndrome
B. Brown Sequard syndrome
C. Anterior cord syndrome
D. Conus medullaris syndrome

Question 138.

The therapist is performing an orthopedic test on a 25-year-old man with the chief complaint of low back pain. The patient has a positive Thomas test. With this information, what might the therapist need to include in the treatment plan?

A. Stretching of the hip abductors
B. Stretching of the hip adductors
C. Stretching of the hip extensors
D. Stretching of the hip flexors

Question 139.

A therapist is performing a chart review and discovers that lab results reveal that the patient has malignant cancer. When evaluating the patient, the therapist is asked by the patient, "Did my lab results come back and is the cancer malignant?" The appropriate response for the therapist is:

A. To tell the patient the truth and contact the social worker to assist in consultation of the family.
B. "It is inappropriate for me to comment on your diagnosis before the doctor has assessed the lab results and spoken to you first."
C. "The results are positive for malignant cancer, but I do not have the training to determine your prognosis."
D. To tell the patient the results are in, but physical therapists are not allowed to speak on this matter.

Question 140.

To facilitate development of a functional tenodesis grip in a patient with spinal cord injury, the treatment plan should include:

A. Stretching of the finger flexors and finger extensors
B. Stretching of the finger flexors
C. Allowing the finger flexors and finger extensors to shorten
D. Allowing the finger flexors to shorten

Question 141.

A 52-year-old man with sciatica presents to outpatient physical therapy. The patient indicates that he is experiencing parasthesia extending to the left ankle and severe lumbar pain. Straight leg-raise test is positive with the left lower extremity. Of the following, which is the most likely source of pain?

A. A lumbar disc with a left posterior herniation or protrusion
B. A lumbar disc with a right posterior herniation or protrusion
C. Piriformis syndrome
D. Sacroiliac joint dysfunction

Question 142.

A patient is scheduled to undergo extremely risky heart surgery. The patient seems really worried. During the treatment session, the patient and family look to the therapist for comfort. Which of the following is an appropriate response from the therapist to the patient?

A. "Don't worry, everything will be okay."
B. "Your physician is the best, and he will take care of you."
C. "I know it must be upsetting to face such a difficult situation. Your family and friends are here to support you."
D. "Try not to worry. Worrying increases your blood pressure and heart rate, which are two factors that need to be stabilized before surgery."

Question 143.

The therapist is ambulating a 42-year-old man who has just received an above-knee prosthesis for the left leg. The therapist notices pistoning of the prosthesis as the patient ambulates. Which of the following is the most probable cause of this deviation?

A. The socket is too small
B. The socket is too large
C. The foot bumper is too soft
D. The foot bumper is too hard

Question 144.

A patient who has suffered a recent fracture of the right tibia and fibula has developed foot drop of the right foot during gait. Which nerve is causing this loss of motor function?

A. Posterior tibial
B. Superficial peroneal
C. Deep peroneal
D. Anterior tibial

Question 145.

A patient is positioned by the therapist with the cervical spine rotated to the right. The patient then extends the neck as the therapist externally rotates and extends the right upper extremity. The patient is then instructed to hold a deep breath. The radial pulse is palpated in the right upper extremity by the therapist. What type of special test is this, and for what condition is it testing?

A. Adson's maneuver—cervical disc herniation
B. Lhermitte's sign—cervical disc herniation
C. Adson's maneuver—thoracic outlet syndrome
D. Lhermitte's sign—thoracic outlet syndrome

Question 146.

A therapist is asked to estimate the percentage of a patient's body that has been burned. The patient is a 32-year-old man of normal size. Burns are located along the entire anterior surface of the face. The patient also burned the entire anterior portion of the right upper extremity in an attempt to guard himself from flames. Using the rule of nines, what percentage of the patient's body is burned?

A. 9%
B. 18%
C. 4.5%
D. 27%

Question 147.

A patient is sitting over the edge of a table and performing active knee extension exercises using an ankle weight as resistance. This exercise demonstrates what class lever?

A. First class
B. Second class
C. Third class
D. Fourth class

Question 148.

A patient is referred to physical therapy services for care of a burn wound on the left foot. The majority of the wound is anesthetic. There is significant eschar formation over the dorsum of the involved foot, and moderate subcutaneous tissue damage is present. What is the most likely classification of this burn?

A. Electrical
B. Superficial partial thickness
C. Deep partial thickness
D. Full thickness

Question 149.

A physical therapy technician calls the therapist immediately to the other side of the outpatient clinic. The therapist discovers a 37-year-old female lying face down on the floor. Which of the following sequence of events is most appropriate for this situation?

A. Have someone call 911, determine unresponsiveness, establish an airway, and assess breathing (look/listen/feel)
B. Determine unresponsiveness, have someone call 911, establish an airway, and assess breathing (look/listen/feel)
C. Have someone call 911, determine unresponsiveness, assess breathing (look/listen/feel), establish an airway
D. Determine unresponsiveness, have someone call 911, assess breathing (look/listen/feel), and establish an airway

Question 150.

The therapist observes a patient with the latter stages of Parkinson's disease during ambulation. Which of the following characteristics is the therapist most likely observing?

A. Shuffling gait
B. Increased step width
C. Difficulty initiating the first steps
D. A and C

Question 151.

A therapist is evaluating the gait pattern of a patient and notes that the pelvis drops inferiorly on the right during the mid-swing phase of the right lower extremity. The patient also leans laterally to the left with the upper trunk during this phase. Which of the following is the most likely cause of this deviation?

A. Weak right gluteus medius
B. Weak right adductor longus
C. Weak left gluteus medius
D. Weak left adductor longus

Question 152.

The therapist is performing an orthopedic test that involves: (1) placing the patient in a sidelying position, (2) placing the superior lower extremity in hip extension and hip abduction, (3) placing the knee of the superior lower extremity in 90° of flexion, and (4) allowing the superior lower extremity to drop into adduction. Failure of the superior lower extremity to drop indicates a tight:

A. Iliopsoas
B. Rectus femoris
C. Iliotibial band
D. Hamstring

Question 153.

An infant with Erb's palsy presents with the involved upper extremity in which of the following positions?

A. Hand supinated and wrist extended
B. Hand supinated and wrist flexed
C. Hand pronated and wrist extended
D. Hand pronated and wrist flexed

Question 154.

A patient is positioned in the supine position. The involved left upper extremity is positioned by the therapist in 90° of shoulder flexion. The therapist applies resistance into shoulder flexion, then extension. No movement takes place. The therapist instructs the patient to "hold" when resistance is applied in both directions. Which of the following proprioceptive neuromuscular facilitation techniques is being used?

A. Repeated contractions
B. Hold-relax
C. Rhythmic stabilization
D. Contract-relax

Question 155.

During a case conference, a respiratory therapist indicates that the patient has a low expiratory reserve volume. What does this mean?

A. The volume of air remaining in the lungs after a full expiration is low
B. The volume of air in a breath during normal breathing is low
C. The volume of air forcefully expired after a forceful inspiration is low
D. The amount of air expired after a resting expiration is low

Question 156.

During the evaluation of an infant, the therapist observes that with passive flexion of the head the infant actively flexes the arms and actively extends the legs. Which of the following reflexes is being observed?

A. Protective extension
B. Optical righting
C. Symmetrical tonic neck
D. Labyrinthine head righting

Question 157.

A patient asks the therapist whether she should be concerned that her 4-month-old infant cannot roll from his back to his stomach. The most appropriate response to the parent is:

A. "This is probably nothing to be concerned about because, although it varies, infants can usually perform this task by 10 months of age"
B. "This is probably nothing to be concerned about because, although it varies, infants can usually perform this task by 5 months of age"
C. "Your infant probably needs further evaluation by a specialist because, although it varies, infants can usually perform this task at 2 months of age"
D. "Your infant probably needs further evaluation by a specialist because, although it varies, infants can usually perform this task at birth"

Question 158.

While evaluating a patient who has just received a new left below-knee prosthesis, the therapist notes that the toe of the prosthesis stays off the floor after heel strike. Which of the following is an unlikely cause of this deviation?

A. The prosthetic foot is set too far anterior
B. The prosthetic foot is set in too much dorsiflexion
C. The heel wedge is too stiff
D. The prosthetic foot is outset too much

Question 159.

A physical therapist receives an order to evaluate a home health patient. The primary nurse states that the patient "may have suffered a stroke because she cannot move the right leg when she stands." The history that the therapist obtains from the patient and family members includes: (1) left total hip replacement 6 months ago, (2) inability to lift the right lower extremity off of the floor in a standing position, (3) recent fall at home 2 nights ago, (4) left lower extremity strength with manual muscle testing in supine is 2+/5 overall, (5) complaints of pain with resisted movement of the left lower extremity, (6) right lower extremity strength is 4+/5 overall, (7) no pain with resisted movements with the right lower extremity, (8) no difference in bilateral upper extremity strength, (9) no decreased sensation, (10) no facial droop, (11) history of dementia but no decreased cognitive ability or speech level as compared with the prior level of function, and (12) independence in ambulation with a standard walker before the recent fall. The therapist's recommendation to the nursing staff should be:

A. The patient should receive physical therapy for strengthening exercises to the right lower extremity with standing exercises and gait training
B. The patient should receive a physician's evaluation for a possible stroke
C. The patient should receive a physician's evaluation for a possible left hip fracture
D. The patient should receive physical therapy for strengthening the left lower extremity and gait training

Question 160.

A physician prescribes isotonic exercises for the left biceps brachii. Which of the following exercises is in compliance with this order?

A. Bicep curls with the patient actively and independently flexing the left elbow using a 5-pound dumbbell as resistance
B. Rhythmic stabilization for the left elbow
C. Elbow flexion at 90° per second with speed controlled by a work simulator
D. None of the above

Question 161.

A diabetic patient is exercising vigorously in an outpatient clinic. The patient informs the therapist that he or she received insulin immediately before the exercise session. If the patient goes into a hypoglycemic coma, which of the following is not a likely sign?

A. Pallor
B. Shallow respiration
C. Bounding pulse
D. Dry skin

Question 162.

A patient has been diagnosed with systemic lupus erythematosus. Which of the following is not a sign of this autoimmune disease?

A. Increased photosensitivity
B. Oral ulcers
C. Butterfly rash
D. Increased number of white blood cells

Question 163.

A physician instructs the therapist to educate a patient about the risk factors of atherosclerosis. Which of the following is the most inappropriate list?

A. Diabetes, male gender, and excessive alcohol
B. Genetic predisposition, smoking, and sedentary lifestyle
C. Stress and inadequate exercise
D. Obesity, smoking, and hypotension

Question 164.

A study of the local population was necessary to determine the need for a new fitness center in the area. The therapists performing the study divided the population by sex and selected a random sample from each group. This is an example of what type of random sample?

A. Systematic random sample
B. Random cluster sample
C. Two stage cluster sample
D. Stratified random sample

Question 165.

A physical therapist instructs a physical therapy assistant to teach a patient how to ascend and descend the front steps of her home. After first exercising the patient at her home, the assistant realizes that, because of her increased size and severe dynamic balance deficits, training on the steps is unsafe at this time. The assistant contacts the therapist by telephone. Which of the following is the best course of action by the therapist?

A. The therapist should instruct the assistant to attempt step training cautiously
B. The therapist should instruct the assistant to recruit the family members to assist with step training
C. The therapist should instruct the assistant to discontinue step training until both of them can be present
D. The therapist should contact the physician and seek further instructions

Question 166.

When reviewing a patient's chart, the therapist determines that the patient has a condition in which the cauda equina is in a fluid-filled sac protruding from the back. What form of spina bifida does the patient most likely have?

A. Meningocele
B. Meningomyelocele
C. Spina bifida occulta
D. None of the above

Question 167.

A 27-year-old woman is referred to a physical therapy clinic with a diagnosis of torticollis. The right sternocleidomastoid is involved. What is the most likely position of the patient's cervical spine?

A. Right lateral cervical flexion and left cervical rotation
B. Right cervical rotation and right lateral cervical flexion
C. Left cervical rotation and left lateral cervical flexion
D. Left lateral cervical flexion and right cervical rotation

Question 168.

During an evaluation, the therapist taps on the flexor retinaculum of the patient's wrist, which causes tingling in the thumb. What test is this? For what condition does it screen?

A. Phalen's test—carpal tunnel
B. Finkelstein test—de Quervain's disease
C. Tinel's sign—de Quervain's disease
D. Tinel's sign—carpal tunnel

Question 169.

Which of the following tissues absorbs the least amount of an ultrasound beam at 1 MHz?

A. Bone
B. Skin
C. Muscle
D. Blood

Question 170.

During the history a 74-year-old woman informs you that she is "taking a heart pill." The patient does not have her medication with her but states that the medication "slows down my heart rate." Which of the following is the most probable medication?

A. Epinephrine
B. Digitalis
C. Quinidine
D. Norepinephrine

Question 171.

A therapist receives an order to evaluate a patient on the telemetry floor of a hospital. The therapist is informed at the nurses' station that an evaluation will not be necessary because the patient went into shock earlier that morning and died. The patient suffered a myocardial infarction earlier, resulting in damage to the left ventricle. Given the above information, what is the most likely type of shock?

A. Vascular shock
B. Anaphylactic shock
C. Toxic shock
D. Cardiogenic shock

Question 172.

A therapist is assessing radial deviation range of motion at the wrist. The correct position of the goniometer should be as follows: the proximal arm aligned with the forearm and the distal arm aligned with the third metacarpal. What should be used as the axis point?

A. Lunate
B. Scaphoid
C. Capitate
D. Triquetrum

Question 173.

Which of the following acts forced all federally supported facilities to increase corridor width to a minimum of 54 inches to accommodate wheelchairs?

A. Americans with Disabilities Act
B. National Healthcare and Resource Development Act
C. Civil Rights Act
D. Older Americans Act (title III)

Question 174.

A therapist is obtaining a subjective history from a new patient diagnosed with right-side hemiplegia. The therapist notes that the patient is able to understand spoken language but unable to speak well. Most of the patient's words are incomprehensible. The patient also has difficulty in naming simple objects. What type of aphasia does the patient most likely have?

A. Anomic aphasia
B. Broca's aphasia
C. Crossed aphasia
D. Wernicke's aphasia

Question 175.

A physician is preparing a patient for an upcoming procedure. The physician explains that the procedure will provide a detailed image that appears to be a slice of the brain. This image is obtained with a highly concentrated x-ray beam. What procedure is the patient scheduled to undergo?

A. Angiogram
B. Magnetic resonance imaging (MRI)
C. Positron emission tomography (PET)
D. Computed tomography (CT)

Question 176.

A patient at an outpatient facility experiences the onset of a grand mal seizure. Which of the following is the most appropriate course of action by the therapist?

A. Assist patient to a lying position, move away close furniture, loosen tight clothes, and prop the patient's mouth open
B. Assist patient to a lying position, move away close furniture, and loosen tight clothes
C. Assist the patient to a seated position, move away close furniture, and loosen tight clothes
D. Assist the patient to a seated position, move away close furniture, loosen tight clothing, and prop the patient's mouth open

Question 177.

A supervisor in an outpatient facility is classified as a McGregor Theory X manager. Which of the following is the most appropriate characterization of the manager's beliefs?

A. Work is natural for most people, workers will use their own self control to accomplish tasks, and workers will accept responsibility for their own actions
B. Workers have low drive, workers are concerned with their own job security, and employees do not like to work
C. Making decisions in the group is the best way to accomplish tasks, and encouraging a long term career for the employee is best
D. There are factors at work that satisfy or dissatisfy an employee

Question 178.

A 3-month-old infant has a heart condition known as tetralogy of Fallot. This condition presents with which of the following signs?

A. Atrial septal defect, pulmonary valve stenosis, aorta abnormally located to the right, and right ventricular hypertrophy
B. Atrial septal defect, pulmonary valve stenosis, aorta abnormally located to the left, and right ventricular hypertrophy
C. Ventricular septal defect, pulmonary valve stenosis, aorta abnormally located to the right, and right ventricular hypertrophy
D. Ventricular septal defect, pulmonary valve stenosis, aorta abnormally located to the right, and left ventricular hypertrophy

Question 179.

Observing a patient in a standing position, the therapist notes that an angulation deformity of the right knee causes it to be located medially in relation to the left hip and left foot. This condition is commonly referred to as:

A. Genu varum
B. Genu valgum
C. Pes cavus
D. None of the above

Question 180.

Which of the following is the most vulnerable position for dislocation of the hip?

A. 30° hip extension, 30° hip adduction, and minimal internal rotation
B. 30° hip flexion, 30° hip adduction, and minimal external rotation
C. 30° hip flexion, 30° hip abduction, and minimal external rotation
D. 30° hip extension, 30° hip abduction , and minimal external rotation

Question 181.

Which of the following articulate with the second cuneiform?

A. Navicular
B. Talus
C. First metatarsal
D. Cuboid

Question 182.

After arriving at the home of a home health patient, the primary nurse informs the therapist that she has activated emergency medical services. The nurse found the patient in what appears to be a diabetic coma. Which of the following is most likely not one of the patient's signs?

A. Skin flush
B. Rapid pulse
C. Weak pulse
D. High blood pressure

Question 183.

Which of the following is the most appropriate orthotic for a patient with excessive foot pronation during static standing?

A. Scaphoid pad
B. Metatarsal pad
C. Metatarsal bar
D. Rocker bar

Question 184.

A patient who suffered a myocardial infarction is participating in an exercise test. The therapist notes ST-segment depression of 1.7 mm on the patient's current rhythm strip. What is the most appropriate course of action?

A. Stop the exercise session immediately and send the patient to the emergency room
B. Continue with the exercise session
C. Contact the patient's cardiologist about continuing exercise
D. Stop the exercise session to take the patient's heart rate and blood pressure

Question 185.

A therapist is instructing a patient in the use of a wrist-driven prehension orthotic. What must be done to achieve opening of the involved hand?

A. Actively extend the wrist
B. Passively extend the wrist
C. Actively flex the wrist
D. Passively flex the wrist

Question 186.

A therapist is scheduled to treat a patient with cerebral palsy who has been classified as a spastic quadriplegic. What type of orthopedic deformity should the therapist expect to see in the patient's feet?

A. Talipes equinovalgus
B. Talipes equinovarus
C. Clubfeet
D. B and C are correct

Question 187.

Which type of atrioventricular (AV) block is present, given the following information about the patient's rhythm strip: P waves are normal and have a QRS complex following, P-R intervals are longer than 0.2 seconds, and the heart rate is 82 beats per minute?

A. First-degree AV block
B. Second-degree AV block—type 1
C. Second-degree AV block—type 2
D. Third-degree AV block

Question 188.

The therapist is treating a patient who received an above-elbow amputation 2 years ago. The prosthesis has a split cable that controls the elbow and the terminal device. With this type of prosthesis, the patient must first lock the elbow to allow the cable to activate the terminal device. This is accomplished with what movements?

A. Extending the humerus and elevating the scapula
B. Extending the humerus and retracting the scapula
C. Extending the humerus and protracting the scapula
D. Extending the humerus and depressing the scapula

Question 189.

A therapist is instructing a physical therapy student in writing a SOAP note. The student has misplaced the following phrase: Patient reports a functional goal of returning to playing baseball in 5 weeks. Where should this phrase be placed in a SOAP note?

A. **S**ubjective
B. **O**bjective
C. **A**ssessment
D. **P**lan

Question 190.

A 32-year-old construction worker fell off a ladder. In his effort to prevent the fall, the worker reached for a beam with his right arm. This motion stretched the brachial plexus, resulting in decreased function in the right arm. Full function returned after 2½ weeks. What is the most likely type of injury?

A. Axonotmesis
B. Neurotmesis
C. Neurapraxia
D. None of the above

Question 191.

A therapist is ordered to evaluate and treat a full-term infant. After reviewing the chart, the therapist discovers that at 1 minute after birth the infant exhibited the following symptoms: bluish color in the body and extremities, heart rate of 85 beats/minute, slow respirations, no response to reflex irritability, and some resistance of the extremities to movement. What was the infant's APGAR score at 1 minute after birth?

A. 1
B. 2
C. 3
D. 4

Question 192.

A therapist is attempting to gain external rotation range of motion in a patient's right shoulder. The therapist decides to use contract-relax-contract antagonist. In what order should the following rotator cuff muscles contract to perform this movement successfully?

A. Infraspinatus—teres minor
B. Subscapularis—supraspinatus
C. Teres minor—infraspinatus
D. Supraspinatus—subscapularis

Question 193.

A therapist is ordered by a physician to treat a patient with congestive heart failure in an outpatient cardiac rehabilitation facility. Which of the following signs and symptoms should the therapist not expect?

A. Stenosis of the mitral valve
B. Orthopnea
C. Decreased preload of the right heart
D. Pulmonary edema

Question 194.

Which of the following is the next response of the leukocytes after emigration into the blood stream in the acute inflammatory stage?

A. Margination
B. Pavementing
C. Adhesion
D. Engulfment

Question 195.

The therapist is treating a patient who recently received a below-knee amputation. The therapist notices in the patient's chart that a psychiatrist has stated that the patient is in the second stage of the grieving process. Which stage of the grieving process is this patient most likely exhibiting?

A. Denial
B. Acceptance
C. Depression
D. Anger

Question 196.

A patient has traumatically dislocated the tibia directly posteriorly during an automobile accident. Which of the following structures is the least likely to be injured?

A. Tibial nerve
B. Popliteal artery
C. Common peroneal nerve
D. Anterior cruciate ligament

Question 197.

The director of a physical therapy facility is in the process of conducting interviews for a staff physical therapist position that will be open in a few weeks. Which of the following questions is inappropriate for the director to ask during the job interview?

A. "What were some of your duties at your previous job?"
B. "Do you have any children?"
C. "What continuing education have you attended within the last year?"
D. "How many years of experience do you have?"

Question 198.

The therapist is assessing a patient's strength in the right shoulder. The patient has 0° of active shoulder abduction in the standing position. In the supine position, the patient has 42° of active shoulder abduction and 175° of pain-free passive shoulder abduction. What is the correct manual muscle testing grade for the patient's shoulder abduction?

A. 3–/5 (fair–).
B. 2+/5 (poor+).
C. 2–/5 (poor–).
D. 1/5 (trace).

Question 199.

A 32-year-old man is referred to physical therapy with the diagnosis of a recent complete anterior cruciate ligament tear. The patient and the physician have decided to avoid surgery as long as possible. The therapist provides the patient with a home exercise program and instructions about activities that will be limited secondary to this diagnosis. Which of the following is the best advice?

A. There are no precautions
B. The patient should avoid all athletic activity for 1 year
C. The patient should avoid all athletic activity until there is a minimum of 20% difference in the bilateral quadriceps muscle as measured isokinetically
D. The patient should wear a brace and compete in only light athletic events

Question 200.

The therapist decides to use electrical stimulation to increase a patient's quadriceps strength. Which of the following is the best protocol?

A. Electrodes placed over the superior/lateral quadriceps and the vastus medialis obliquus—stimulation on for 15 seconds, then off for 15 seconds
B. Electrodes over the femoral nerve in the proximal quadriceps and the vastus medialis obliquus—stimulation on for 50 seconds, then off for 10 seconds
C. Electrodes over the vastus medialis obliquus and superior/lateral quadriceps—stimulation frequency set between 50–80 hertz, pps
D. Electrodes over the femoral nerve in the proximal quadriceps and the vastus medialis obliquus—stimulation frequency set between 50–80 hertz, pps

Question 201.

A therapist is treating a patient with an injury at the T8 level and compromised function of the diaphragm. If no abdominal binder is available, what is the most likely position of comfort to allow him to breathe most efficiently?

A. Sitting position
B. Semi-Fowler's position
C. Upright standing position using a tilt table
D. Supine

Question 202.

A therapist is assisting a patient with an injury at the C5 level in performing an effective cough. The patient has experienced significant neurologic damage and is unable to perform an independent, effective cough. If the patient is in supine position, which of the following methods is most likely to produce an effective cough?

A. The therapist places the heel of one hand just above the xiphoid process, instructs the patient to take a deep breath while pressing down moderately on the sternum, and instructs the patient to cough.
B. The therapist places the heel of one hand, reinforced with the other hand, just above the xiphoid process; instructs the patient to take a deep breath; instructs the patient to hold the breath; and presses moderately as the patient coughs.
C. The therapist places the heel of one hand on the area just above the umbilicus, instructs the patient to take a deep breath, applies moderate pressure, and releases pressure just before the patient attempts to cough.
D. The therapist places the heel of one hand just above the umbilicus, instructs the patient to take a deep breath, and applies moderate pressure as the patient is instructed to cough.

Question 203.

A patient with dysarthria and dysphagia is being treated by physical and speech therapy services. The physical therapist can assist the patient in which of the following ways?

A. Provide posture control exercises; teach the patient swallowing techniques of thin liquids; provide facial musculature exercises; provide good verbal interaction.
B. Teach the patient to have good eye contact; provide facial musculature exercises; teach increased head and trunk control.
C. Provide posture control exercises; provide multiple sources of stimuli during exercise sessions; teach the patient swallowing techniques of thin liquids; teach the patient swallowing techniques for prescribed medications in capsular form.
D. None of the above lists is completely correct.

Question 204.

A 30-year-old man is referred to physical therapy after a recent motor vehicle accident that resulted in total loss of motor control of both legs. Trunk and bilateral upper extremity control allows independent sitting at bedside. The patient is to be discharged from the hospital and will return home a few hours after the physical therapy session. The therapist notices, from the history in the chart, that the patient lives alone and has little or no outside support from family members. The patient also suffers from severe obesity. The therapist decides to practice a transfer from the bed to the wheelchair. Which assistive device should the therapist use for this transfer attempt?

A. Hoyer lift (pneumatic lift)
B. Sliding board
C. Geriatric chair (using a slide sheet transfer)
D. Trapeze bar

Question 205.

A therapist should consider using a form of treatment other than moist heat application on the posterior lumbar region of all of the following patients except:

A. Patient with a history of hemophilia
B. Patient with a history of malignant cancer under the site of heat application
C. Patient with a history of Raynaud's phenomenon
D. Patient with a history including many years of steroid therapy

Question 206.

A 50-year-old woman has been receiving treatment in the hospital for increased edema in the right upper extremity. The therapist has treated the patient for the past 3 weeks with an intermittent compression pump equipped with a multicompartment compression sleeve. The patient's average blood pressure is 135/80 mmHg. The daily sessions are 3 hours in duration. The pump is set at 50 mmHg, 40 mmHg, and 30 mmHg (distal to proximal) for 30 seconds, on and off for 15 seconds. The therapist decides to change the parameters. Of the following changes, which is the most likely to increase the efficiency of treatment?

A. Place the patient in a seated position with the right upper extremity in a dependent position versus supine and elevated
B. Increase the maximal pressure from 50 mmHg to 60 mmHg
C. Change the on/off time to 15 seconds on and 45 seconds off
D. Equalize the sleeve compartments versus having greater pressure distally

Question 207.

A therapist chose to work with her patient using fluidotherapy rather than paraffin wax. The patient has lack of range of motion and also needs to decrease hypersensitivity. There are no open wounds on the hand to be treated. Which of the following would not be an advantage of using fluidotherapy vs. paraffin wax in the above scenario?

A. The therapist can assist range of motion manually while the patient has his hand in the fluidotherapy and not while in the paraffin wax
B. The fluidotherapy can be used to assist in desensitation by adjusting air intensity
C. The fluidotherapy can be provided at the same time as dynamic splinting, and this cannot be done while in paraffin wax
D. The fingers can be bound, to assist gaining finger flexion, with tape while in fluidotherapy and not in paraffin wax

Question 208.

The terms below refer to properties of water that make hydrotherapy valuable to a variety of patient populations. Match the following terms with the statement that best relates to each term.

1 • Viscosity
2 • Buoyancy
3 • Relative density
4 • Hydrostatic pressure
a • This property can assist in prevention of blood pooling in the lower extremities of a patient in the pool above waist level.
b • This property makes it harder to walk faster through water.
c • A person with a higher amount of body fat can float more easily than a lean person because of this property.
d • This property makes it easier to move a body part to the surface of the water and harder to move a part away from the surface.

A. 1-b, 2-c, 3-d, 4-a
B. 1-b, 2-d, 3-c, 4-a
C. 1-c, 2-b, 3-a, 4-d
D. 1-a, 2-c, 3-b, 4-d

Question 209.

Which of the following statements is false about treatment with infrared lamps?

A. Near infrared heats deeper than far infrared.
B. Infrared lamps heat both sides of an extremity at one time.
C. The therapist can change the intensity of the heat by changing the angle between the beam and the body part being treated.
D. The therapist can change the intensity by placing the lamp closer to the part being treated.

Question 210.

A patient is referred to physical therapy because of hypertension. The physician has ordered relaxation training. The therapist first chooses to instruct the patient in the technique of diaphragmatic breathing. Which of the below is the correct set of instructions?

A. Slow breathing rate to 8–12 breaths per minute, increase movement of the upper chest, and decrease movement in the abdominal region
B. Slow breathing rate to 12–16 breaths per minute, increase movement of the abdominal region, and decrease movement in the upper chest
C. Slow breathing rate to 8–12 breaths per minute, increase movement of the abdominal region, and decrease movement in the upper chest
D. Slow breathing rate to 12–16 breaths per minute, increase movement of the upper chest, and decrease movement in the abdominal region

Question 211.

An acute-care physical therapist is ordered to evaluate and treat a patient who has suffered a right hip fracture in a recent fall. During the evaluation, the family informs the therapist that the patient suffered a stroke approximately 1 week before the fall. The patient's chart has no record of the recent stroke. What should the physical therapist do first?

A. Immediately call the referring physician and request a magnetic resonance scan
B. Evaluate and treat the patient as ordered
C. Immediately call the referring physician and request a computed tomography scan
D. Immediately call the referring physician for an occupational therapy referral

Question 212.

A physical therapist in an outpatient clinic is urgently called into a room to assist an infant who is unconscious and not breathing. The therapist opens the airway of the infant and attempts ventilation. The breaths do not make the chest rise. After the infant's head is repositioned, the breaths still do not cause the chest to move. What should the therapist do next?

A. Give five back blows
B. Look into the throat for a foreign body
C. Have someone call 911
D. Perform a blind finger sweep of the throat

Question 213.

A physical therapist is assessing a 40-year-old man's balance and coordination. The following instructions are given to the patient: "Stand normally, with your eyes open. After fifteen seconds, close your eyes and maintain a normal standing posture." Several seconds after closing his eyes, the patient nearly falls. What type of test did the patient fail?

A. Nonequilibrium test
B. Equilibrium test
C. Romberg test
D. B and C

Question 214.

A patient presents to an outpatient clinic with a diagnosis of reflex sympathetic dystrophy (RSD) of the left upper extremity. The physician's order is to evaluate and treat. While obtaining a subjective history, the therapist is informed that the patient has a long-standing diagnosis of carpal tunnel syndrome. Left upper extremity signs and symptoms include constant burning pain, abnormal fast hair and nail growth, decreased range of motion, and increased sensitivity to pain and/or light touch. Given the above information, the patient is most likely in what stage of RSD?

A. Acute
B. Dystrophic
C. Atrophic
D. Chronic

Question 215.

A physician has ordered a physical therapist to treat a patient with chronic low back pain. The order is to "increase gluteal muscle function by decreasing trigger points in the quadratus lumborum." What is the first technique that should be used by the physical therapist?

A. Isometric gluteal strengthening
B. Posture program
C. Soft tissue massage
D. Muscle reeducation

Question 216.

A physical therapist is ordered to evaluate a 65-year-old woman who has suffered a recent stroke. The occupational therapist informs the physical therapist that the patient has apraxia. She cannot brush her teeth on command. However, she can point out the toothbrush and verbalize the purpose of the brush. From this information, what sort of apraxia does this patient have? How should the physical therapist approach treatment?

A. Ideomotor apraxia. The physical therapist should speak in short, concise sentences.
B. Ideational apraxia. The physical therapist should always give the patient 3-step commands.
C. Ideomotor apraxia. The physical therapist should always give the patient 3-step commands.
D. Ideational apraxia. The physical therapist should speak in short, concise sentences.

Question 217.

A 60-year-old woman who has suffered a recent stroke has right-side homonymous hemianopsia. Which of the following statements is true about placement of eating utensils in early rehabilitation?

A. The utensils should be placed on the left side of the plate
B. The utensils should be placed on the right side of the plate
C. The utensils should be placed on both sides of the plate
D. The plate and utensils should be placed slightly to the right

Question 218.

The physical therapist has just given the patient a custom wheelchair. The patient has a long-standing history of hamstring contractures resulting in fixation of the knees into 60° of flexion. The patient is also prone to develop decubitus ulcers. Which of the following is incorrect advice to give the family and patient?

A. Keep the patient's buttocks clean and dry
B. Make sure that the wheelchair cushion is always in the wheelchair seat
C. Keep the leg rests of the wheelchair fully elevated
D. Never transfer using a sliding board from one surface to another

Question 219.

Which of the following circumstances would normally decrease body temperature in a healthy person?

A. Exercising on a treadmill
B. Pregnancy
C. Normal ovulation
D. Reaching age of 65 years or older

Question 220.

Which of the following statements is false about cardiovascular response to exercise in trained and/or sedentary patients?

A. If exercise intensities are equal, the sedentary patient's heart rate will increase faster than the trained patient's heart rate
B. Cardiovascular response to increased workload will increase at the same rate for sedentary as it will for trained patients
C. Trained patients will have a larger stroke volume during exercise
D. The sedentary patient will reach anaerobic threshold faster than the trained patient, if workloads are equal

Question 221.

Use of short-wave diathermy and microwave diathermy is not contraindicated in which of the following conditions?

A. On a patient who has a pacemaker
B. Over the site of a metal implant
C. On a patient who has hemophilia
D. Using pulsed short-wave over an acute injury

Question 222.

A therapist is treating a 35-year-old man who has suffered loss of motor control in the right lower extremity due to peripheral neuropathy. The therapist applies biofeedback electrodes to the right quadricep in an effort to increase control and strength of this muscle group. The biofeedback can help achieve this goal in all of the following ways except:

A. Providing visual input for the patient to know how hard he is contracting the right quadricep
B. Assisting the patient in recruitment of more motor units in the right quadricep
C. Providing a measure of torque in the right quadricep
D. Providing the therapist input on the patient's ability and effort in contracting the right quadricep

Question 223.

When using electrical stimulation with a unit that plugs into the wall, the therapist must take many different safety precautions. Which of the following precautions probably would not increase safety to the patient and therapist?

A. Never placing the unit in close proximity to water pipes while treating the patient
B. Never using an extension cord when using a plug-in unit
C. Always adjusting the intensity of stimulation during the off portion of the cycle
D. Both A and C are measures that are not likely to increase safety

Question 224.

A patient is receiving electrical stimulation for muscle strengthening of the left quadricep. One electrode from one lead wire, 4×4 inches in size, is placed on the anterior proximal portion of the left quadricep. Each of two other electrodes from one lead wire are 2×2 inches in size. One of the electrodes is placed on the inferior medial side of the left quadricep and one on the inferior lateral side of the left quadricep. This is an example of what type of electrode configuration?

A. Monopolar
B. Bipolar
C. Tripolar
D. Quadripolar

Question 225.

A 60-year-old woman is referred to outpatient physical therapy services for rehabilitation after receiving a left total knee replacement 4 weeks ago. The patient is currently ambulating with a standard walker with a severely antalgic gait pattern. Before the recent surgery the patient was ambulating independently without an assistive device. Left knee flexion was measured in the initial evaluation and found to be 85° actively and 94° passively. The patient also lacked 10° of full passive extension and 17° of full active extension. Which of the following does the therapist need to first address?

A. Lack of passive left knee flexion
B. Lack of passive left knee extension
C. Lack of active left knee extension
D. Ability to ambulate with a lesser assistive device

Question 226.

In comparing the use of cold pack and hot pack treatments, which of the following statements is false?

A. Cold packs penetrate more deeply than hot packs
B. Cold increases the viscosity of fluid and heat decreases the viscosity of fluid
C. Cold decreases spasm by decreasing sensitivity to muscle spindles and heat decreases spasm by decreasing nerve conduction velocity
D. Cold decreases the rate of oxygen uptake, and heat increases the rate of oxygen uptake

Question 227.

A home health physical therapist is sent to evaluate a 56-year-old man who has suffered a recent stroke. The patient is sitting in a lift chair, accompanied by his 14-year-old nephew. He seems confused several times throughout the evaluation. The nephew is unable to assist in clarifying much of the subjective history. The patient reports to the therapist that he is independent in ambulation with a standard walker as an assistive device and in all transfers without an assistive device. Based on the above information, which of the following sequence of events, chosen by the therapist, is in the correct order?

A. Ambulate with the standard walker with the wheelchair in close proximity; transfer sit to stand in front of the wheelchair; transfer wheelchair to bed; assess range of motion and strength of all extremities in supine position
B. Ambulate with the standard walker with the wheelchair in close proximity; transfer wheelchair to bed; assess range of motion and strength of all extremities in supine position; transfer sit to stand at bedside
C. Assess range of motion and strength of all extremities in the lift chair; transfer sit to stand in front of the lift chair; ambulate with the standard walker with the wheelchair in close proximity; transfer wheelchair to bed
D. Assess range of motion and strength of all extremities in the lift chair; ambulate with the standard walker with the wheelchair in close proximity; transfer sit to stand in front of the wheelchair; transfer wheelchair to bed

Question 228.

A therapist is evaluating a patient with poor motor coordination. The therapist observes that when the patient is standing erect and still, she does not respond appropriately when correcting a backward sway of the body. With the body in a fully erect position a slight backward sway should be corrected by the body firing specific muscles in a specific order. Which list is the correct firing order?

A. Bilateral abdominals, bilateral quadriceps, bilateral tibialis anterior
B. Bilateral abdominals, bilateral tibialis anterior, bilateral quadriceps
C. Bilateral tibialis anterior, bilateral abdominals, bilateral quadriceps
D. Bilateral tibialis anterior, bilateral quadriceps, bilateral abdominals

Question 229.

A therapist is assessing a patient's ability to perform basic activities of daily living. The assessment tool chosen by the therapist measures bathing, toileting, dressing, transfers, continence, and feeding. The tool does not assess the patient's ability to maneuver in a wheelchair. The therapist is using which of the following tests?

A. Barthel Index
B. Katz Index of Activities of Daily Living
C. Kenny Self-Care Evaluation
D. Functional Status Index

Question 230.

A physical therapist is performing electromyographic testing. During a maximal output test of the patient's quadricep muscle, 25% of the motor unit action potential is polyphasic. What is the significance of this finding?

A. It is normal in the quadricep.
B. It is normal in the triceps brachii, not in the quadricep.
C. It is normal in the biceps brachii, not in the quadricep.
D. It is abnormal in any muscle.

Question 231.

A physical therapist is ordered to evaluate a patient in the late stages of amyotrophic lateral sclerosis. In the patient's chart is an electromyography report and nerve conduction velocity test. What should the physical therapist not expect to find in these test results?

A. Fibrillation potentials
B. Polyphasic motor unit potentials
C. Decreased sensory evoked potentials
D. A and B only

Question 232.

A 27-year-old man with a diagnosis of incomplete spinal cord injury at the L4 level is being evaluated by a physical therapist. The patient is nearing discharge from the rehabilitation unit. Manual muscle testing reveals the following: right hip flexion = 4/5, right hip adduction = 5/5, right knee flexion = 2/5, right knee extension = 3+/5, right ankle plantarflexion = 1/5, and right ankle dorsiflexion = 2-/5; left hip flexion = 4+/5, left hip adduction = 4+/5, left knee flexion = 2+/5, left knee extension = 3+/5, left ankle plantarflexion = 2-/5, and left ankle dorsiflexion = 2-/5. What is the appropriate orthotic for this patient? What is his most likely functional outcome?

A. Hip-knee-ankle-foot orthosis (HKAFO) with forearm crutches—household ambulator.
B. Knee-ankle-foot orthosis (KAFO) with forearm crutches—household ambulator.
C. KAFO with forearm crutches—functional ambulator.
D. HKAFO with forearm crutches—functional ambulator.

Question 233.

Which of the following should a therapist evaluate first when performing a job-site analysis?

A. Job description and duties
B. Bathroom accessibility
C. Lighting conditions
D. Parking conditions

Question 234.

A physical therapist is treating a patient with balance deficits. During treatment the physical therapist notes that large-amplitude changes in center of mass cause the patient to lose balance. The patient, however, can accurately compensate for small changes nearly every time a change is introduced. What muscles most likely need to be strengthened to help alleviate this dysfunction?

A. Tibialis anterior, gastrocnemius
B. Peroneus longus/brevis, tibialis posterior
C. Rectus abdominis, erector spinea
D. Iliopsoas, gluteus maximus

Question 235.

A physical therapist is treating a patient who is participating in cardiac rehabilitation. Because the patient complains of chest pain, the therapist attempts to assess heart sounds with a stethoscope. Which of the following is true about the first sound during auscultation of the heart?

A. The first sound is of the closure of the aortic and pulmonic valves
B. The first sound is of the closure of the mitral and tricuspid valves
C. The first sound is of the beginning of ventricular systole
D. B and C

Question 236.

A 15-year-old girl with no reports of trauma or radiculopathy presents to an outpatient physical therapy clinic with complaints of low back pain. The physical therapist decides to measure leg length of each side from the anterior superior iliac spine (ASIS) to the medial malleolus. The measurements are equal. However, when measurements are taken from the umbilicus to the medial malleolus, the right lower extremity is 2.5 cm longer than the left lower extremity. Based on the above information, which of the following would most directly address the source of this patient's problem?

A. Ask the patient if she has ever had a femur fracture
B. Ask the patient if she has ever been diagnosed with cerebral palsy or avascular necrosis
C. Ask the patient if she has ever been diagnosed with scoliosis
D. Ask the patient to perform active motion to assess lumbar range of motion

Question 237.

How often does the Joint Commission on Accreditation of Healthcare Organizations (JCAHO) require that all electrical equipment in hospitals be inspected?

A. Every 3 months
B. Every 6 months
C. Every 12 months
D. Every 3 years

Question 238.

A physical therapist is setting up a portable whirlpool unit in the room of a severely immobile patient. What is the most important task of the physical therapist before the patient is placed in the whirlpool?

A. Check for a ground fault circuit interruption outlet
B. Check to make sure the water temperature is below 110°
C. Make sure the whirlpool agitator is immersed in the water
D. Obtain the appropriate assistance to perform a transfer

Question 239.

A 37-year-old man fell and struck his left temple area on the corner of a mat table. He begins to bleed profusely but remains conscious and alert. Attempts to stop blood flow with direct pressure to the area of the injury are unsuccessful. Of the following, which is an additional area to which pressure should be applied to stop bleeding?

A. Left parietal bone one inch posterior to the ear
B. Left temporal bone just anterior to the ear
C. Zygomatic arch of the frontal bone
D. Zygomatic arch superior to the mastoid process

Question 240.

A physical therapist is ordered to provide gait training for an 18-year-old girl who received a partial medial meniscectomy of the right knee one day earlier. The patient was independent in ambulation without an assistive device before surgery and has no cognitive deficits. The patient's weight-bearing status is currently partial weight-bearing on the involved lower extremity. Which of the following is the most appropriate assistive device and gait pattern?

A. Crutches, three-point gait pattern
B. Standard walker, three-point gait pattern
C. Standard walker, four-point gait pattern
D. Crutches, swing-to gait pattern

Question 241.

A physical therapist is treating a 72-year-old woman with a diagnosis of Parkinson's disease 3 times/week at an outpatient facility. The patient is taking 500 mg/day of a medication designed to decrease spasticity. The therapist notices that the patient is performing well on certain days and poorly on others. Which of the following ways can the therapist possibly improve the patient's performance on the days when she performs poorly?

A. The therapist can encourage the patient to increase her daily dosage of medication to 600 mg/day on the days she usually performs poorly
B. The therapist can encourage the patient to decrease her daily dosage of medication to 400 mg/day on the days she usually performs poorly
C. The therapist can schedule sessions so that there are fewer sessions on the days the patient usually performs poorly
D. The therapist can call the physician and recommend another medication

Question 242.

A patient is receiving crutch training 1 day after a right knee arthroscopic surgery. The patient's weight-bearing status is toe-touch weight-bearing on the right lower extremity. The therapist first chooses to instruct the patient how to perform a correct sit to stand transfer. Which of the following is the most correct set of instructions?

A. (1) Slide forward to the edge of the chair; (2) put both the crutches in front of you and hold both grips together with the right hand; (3) press on the left arm rest with the left hand and the grips with the right hand; (4) lean forward; (5) stand up, placing your weight on the left lower extremity; (6) place one crutch slowly under the left arm, then under the right arm.

B. (1) Slide forward; (2) put one crutch in each hand, holding the grips; (3) place crutches in a vertical position; (4) press down on the grips; (5) stand up, placing more weight on the left lower extremity.

C. (1) Slide forward to the edge of the chair; (2) put both the crutches in front of you and hold both grips together with the left hand; (3) press on the right arm rest with the right hand and the grips with the left hand; (4) lean forward; (5) stand up placing your weight on the left lower extremity; (6) place one crutch slowly under the right arm, then under the left arm.

D. (1) Place crutches in close proximity; (2) slide forward; (3) place hands on the arm rests; (4) press down and stand up; (5) place weight on the left lower extremity; (6) reach slowly for the crutches and place under the axilla.

Question 243.

A physical therapist is asked by a coworker to finish evaluating a patient because an emergency requires the therapist to leave. The coworker agrees and resumes the examination. The first therapist left notes titled, "sensory assessment." Two wooden blocks identical in appearance but 1 pound different in weight are on the table in front of the patient. What test was the prior therapist most likely performing?

A. Barognosis test
B. Stereognosis test
C. Graphesthesia test
D. Texture recognition

Question 244.

A therapist places a pen in front of a patient and asks him to pick it up and hold it as he normally would to write. The patient picks the pen up and holds it between the pad of the thumb and the middle and the index fingers. What type of grasp or prehension is the patient using?

A. Palmar prehension
B. Fingertip prehension
C. Lateral prehension
D. Hook grasp

Question 245.

A therapist is sent to the intensive care unit to evaluate a patient who has suffered a severe recent head injury. While reviewing the patient's chart, he discovers that the patient exhibits decerebrate rigidity. The therapist is likely to find this patient in which of the following positions?

A. The patient will be positioned with all extremities extended and the wrist and fingers flexed
B. The patient will be positioned with the upper extremities flexed, the lower extremities hyperextended, and the fingers tightly flexed
C. The patient will be positioned with all extremities flexed and the wrist and fingers extended
D. The patient will be positioned with the upper extremities extended, the lower extremities flexed, and the fingers hyperextended

Question 246.

A therapist is preparing a poster that will clarify some of the data in an inservice presentation. The poster reflects the mode, median, and mean of a set of data. The data consist of the numbers 2, 2, 4, 9, and 13. If presented in the above order (mode, median, mean), which of the following is the correct list of answers calculated from the data?

A. 4, 2, 6
B. 2, 4, 6
C. 6, 2, 4
D. 6, 4, 2

Question 247.

A patient with a spinal cord injury is being treated by physical therapy in an acute rehabilitation setting. The patient has been involved in a motor vehicle accident that resulted in a complete C8 spinal cord lesion. The patient is a 20-year-old man who has expressed concern to the therapist about his future sexual function. Which of the following is the most correct information to convey to this patient?

A. Psychogenic erection is possible, reflexogenic erection is not possible, and ejaculation is possible
B. Psychogenic erection is not possible, reflexogenic erection is not possible, and ejaculation is not possible
C. Psychogenic erection is possible, reflexogenic erection is possible, and ejaculation is possible
D. Psychogenic erection is not possible, reflexogenic erection is possible, and ejaculation is not possible

Question 248.

A therapist is treating a patient with cystic fibrosis who has just walked 75 feet before experiencing significant breathing difficulties. In an effort to assist the patient in regaining her normal breathing rate, the therapist gives a set of instructions. Which of the following set of instructions is appropriate?

A. "Take a slow deep breath through pursed lips and exhale slowly through your nose only"
B. "Take small breaths through your nose only and exhale quickly through pursed lips"
C. "Breath in through your nose and exhale slowly through pursed lips"
D. "Breath in through pursed lips and breath out slowly through pursed lips"

Question 249.

A therapist is massaging the upper trapezius of a patient. One of the techniques involves lifting and kneading of the tissues. What is the correct name of this technique?

A. Tapotement massage
B. Effleurage massage
C. Petrissage massage
D. Friction massage

Question 250.

A therapist is assessing a patient in an attempt to discover the source of her pain. She positions the patient's cervical spine in different directions in an attempt to elicit the patient's symptoms. In one such direction, the patient reports return of symptoms, including pain located at the right posterior scapular region, which extends down the posterior side of the right upper extremity to the ends of the fingers, and tingling in the second, third, and fourth digits. The patient also indicates that she often has a decrease in sensation on the dorsal side of the second and third digits. She also has noticeable weakness in the right triceps. Which nerve root is most likely involved?

A. Fourth cervical root
B. Fifth cervical root
C. Sixth cervical root
D. Seventh cervical root

Question 251.

A patient is being treated with iontophoresis, driving dexamethasone, for inflammation around the lateral epicondyle of the left elbow. The therapist is careful when setting the parameters and with cleaning the site of electrode application to prevent a possible blister. This possibility is not as strong with some other forms of electrical stimulation, but with iontophoresis using a form of _____, precautions must be taken to ensure that the patient does not receive a mild burn or blister during the treatment session. Fill in the blank.

A. Alternating current
B. Direct current
C. Pulsed current
D. Trancutaneous electrical nerve stimulation

Question 252.

A physical therapist is beginning the evaluation of a patient with AIDS. The patient was admitted to the acute floor of the hospital on the previous night after receiving a right total hip replacement. The physician has ordered gait training and a dressing change of the surgical site. Of the following precautions, which is the least necessary?

A. Mask
B. Gloves
C. Handwashing
D. Gown

Question 253.

An outpatient physical therapist notices that a large number of patients with impingement of the rotator cuff have been treated in the past 6 months. The clinic finds that most patients are employed at a new auto manufacturing plant. The therapist is invited to the plant to perform an ergonomic assessment and finds that a certain number of the employees must work with their shoulders at 120° of flexion 6–8 hours/day. Which of the following recommendations would decrease the frequency of injury?

A. Provide the employees with a step stool to perform their tasks
B. Raise the employees' work surface
C. Adjust their tasks so that overhead activities are performed with palm of the hand downward
D. A and B are correct

Question 254.

A physical therapist is treating a 17-year-old boy with an incomplete T11 spinal cord injury. The patient was treated for 2 months in the rehabilitation unit of the hospital before beginning outpatient physical therapy. He is currently ambulating with a standard walker with maximal assist of two. The therapist sets an initial long-term goal of "ambulation with a standard walker with minimum assist of 1 for a distance of 50 feet, with no loss of balance, on a level surface—in 8 weeks." If the patient achieves the long-term goal in 4 weeks, which of the following courses of action should be taken by the therapist?

A. Discharge the patient secondary to completion of goals
B. Set another long-term goal regarding ambulation and continue treatment
C. Return the patient to the rehabilitation unit of the hospital for more intensive treatment
D. Call the patient's physician and ask for further instructions

Question 255.

A physical therapist is ordered to evaluate a 74-year-old man who has suffered a recent stroke. The therapist performs a chart review before performing the evaluation. Which of the following is of the least importance to the physical therapist in assessing the patient's chart?

A. Nursing assessment
B. Physician's orders/notes
C. Respiratory assessment
D. Dietary assessment

Question 256.

A 47-year-old man with end-stage renal disease arrives at an outpatient facility. He has a physician's order to evaluate and treat 3 times/week for 4 weeks secondary to lower extremity weakness. The patient also attends dialysis 3 times/week. If the clinic is open Monday through Friday, which of the following schedule is appropriate?

A. On the days that the patient has dialysis, schedule the therapy session before the dialysis appointment
B. On the days that the patient has dialysis, schedule the therapy session after the dialysis appointment
C. Contact the physician and obtain a new order to decrease the frequency to 2 times/week
D. A and C are correct

Question 257.

A physical therapist is performing a functional capacity evaluation on a patient with a L4–L5 herniated disc. Part of the evaluation consists of performing floor to waist lifts using 30 pounds as resistance. During the first trial, the physical therapist notices that patient exhibits decreased anterior pelvic tilt. What should the physical therapist do during the second trial?

A. Correct the deviation verbally before the lift
B. Correct the deviation with manual contact during the lift
C. Correct the deviation both verbally and manually during the lift
D. None of the above

Question 258.

A 20-year-old man with anterior cruciate ligament reconstruction with allograft presents to an outpatient physical therapy clinic. The patient's surgery was 5 days ago. The patient is independent in ambulation with crutches. He also currently has 53° of active knee flexion and 67° of passive knee flexion and lacks 10° of full knee extension actively and 5° passively. What is the most significant deficit on which the physical therapist should focus treatment?

A. Lack of active knee extension
B. Lack of passive knee extension
C. Lack of active knee flexion
D. Lack of passive knee flexion

Question 259.

A physical therapist is ordered to evaluate and treat in the acute setting a patient who received a left total knee replacement 1 day ago. Before surgery, the patient was independent in all activities of daily living, transfers, and ambulation with an assistive device. The family reports that ambulation was slow and guarded because of knee pain. The physician's orders are to ambulate with partial weight-bearing on the left lower extremity and to increase strength/range of motion. At this point, bed-to-wheelchair transfers, sit-to-stand transfers, and wheelchair-to-toilet transfers require the minimal assistance of one person. The left knee has 63° of active flexion and 77° of passive flexion. The left knee also lacks 7° of full extension actively and 3° passively. Right hip strength is recorded as follows: hip flexion and abduction = 4+/5, hip adduction and extension = 5/5, knee flexion = 4+/5, knee extension = 5/5, ankle plantarflexion = 4+/5, and dorsiflexion = 5/5. Left lower extremity strength is recorded as follows: hip flexion = 3/5, hip abduction and adduction = 3+/5, hip extension =3/5, knee flexion and extension = 3-/5, ankle dorsiflexion = 3+/5, and plantarflexion = 3+/5. The patient is currently able to ambulate 30 feet × 2 with a standard walker and minimal assist of one person on level surfaces. She also ambulates with a flexed knee throughout the gait cycle. According to the physician, she most likely will be discharged to home (with home health services), where she lives alone, within the next 2–3 days. Of the choices below, which is the most important long-term goal in the acute setting?

A. In three days the patient will be independent in all transfers
B. In three days the patient will ambulate with a quad cane independently, with no gait deviations, on level surfaces 50 feet × 3
C. In three days the patient will increase all left lower extremity manual muscle testing grades by one half grade
D. In three days the patient will have active left knee range of motion from 0 to 90° and passive range of motion from 0 to 95°

Question 260.

A physical therapist is in a rehabilitation team meeting about a 58-year-old man with Parkinson's disease. The physician notes that the patient's recent decrease in level of function may be caused by long-term use of a certain drug. The physician plans to take the patient off of the medication for 2 weeks. Which of the following medications is the patient probably taking?

A. Cardizem
B. Cortisone
C. Epinephrine
D. Levodopa

Question 261.

A physical therapist is reviewing the chart of a 49-year-old woman who recently suffered a myocardial infarction. The lab reports reveal that this particular patient has a hematocrit of 41%. How should the therapist proceed?

A. Continue with the evaluation and treatment
B. Do not perform this evaluation due to the hematocrit level
C. Inform nursing of this lab report
D. Check nursing notes to determine the last time the patient received a beta-blocker

Question 262.

A physical therapist is treating a 34-year-old woman with lumbar muscle spasms. Part of the patient's treatment involves receiving instruction on correct sleeping positions. Which of the following would be most comfortable?

A. Supine with no pillows under the head or extremities
B. Prone with a pillow under the head only
C. Sidelying with a pillow between flexed knees
D. A and C are equally correct

Question 263.

The physical therapist is reading the physician's interpretation of an x-ray that was taken of the left humerus of a 7-year-old patient. The physician notes in the report the presence of an incomplete fracture on the convex side of the humerus. Which type of fracture is the physician describing?

A. Comminuted
B. Avulsion
C. Greenstick
D. Segmental

Question 264.

A patient is referred to physical therapy with a history of temporomandibular joint pain. The therapist notices that the patient is having difficulty closing his mouth against minimal resistance. With this information, which of the following muscles would not be a target for strengthening exercise to correct this deficit?

A. Medial pterygoid muscle
B. Temporalis
C. Masseter
D. Lateral pterygoid muscle

Question 265.

An infant is being examined by a physical therapist. The therapist is resisting movement of the right upper extremity and notices involuntary movement of the left upper extremity. Which of the following is displayed by the infant?

A. Landau reaction
B. Startle reflex
C. Moro reflex
D. Associated reaction

Question 266.

A therapist is evaluating an infant with the mother present. The therapist suddenly seems to temporarily lose grip of the infant, causing him to be startled and begin to cry. The infant's mother is noticeably upset but is reassured that startling the infant was part of the assessment. Which of the following may the therapist have been assessing?

A. Landau response
B. Symmetric tonic neck reflex
C. Labyrinthine head righting
D. Moro reflex

Question 267.

A 25-year-old man suffered C4 quadriplegia in a motor vehicle accident. The injury is acute, and the patient is beginning to work on increasing upright tolerance in the sitting position with an abdominal binder. He is looking to the therapist for encouragement. The therapist is attempting to convey realistic long-term goals for self-care ability and overall mobility. Of the below listed goals, what can this patient reasonably expect at his highest level of function in the future?

A. Transfer from wheelchair to bed independently with a sliding board
B. Use of a power wheelchair
C. Independent feeding without an assistive device
D. Donning a shirt independently and pants with minimal assistance

Question 268.

A 17-year-old boy presents to therapy after being involved in a motor vehicle accident resulting in C7 quadriplegia. The therapist is setting long-term goals for the patient. Which of the following goals represents the most reasonable and highest level of function that the patient should achieve?

A. Use of a wheelchair with power hand controls on even terrain
B. Negotiation of uneven terrain with a manual wheelchair
C. Ambulation for short distances on level surfaces with knee-ankle-foot orthoses
D. Use of a power wheelchair with head or chin controls on even surfaces

Question 269.

A therapist is treating a patient with spinal cord injury. The therapist is discharging the patient after completion of all physical therapy goals. One of the completed long-term goals involved the ability to dress and bathe independently with assistive devices. This would be a most challenging but obtainable goal for which of the following?

A. C5 quadriplegia
B. C7 quadriplegia
C. T1 paraplegia
D. C4 quadriplegia

Question 270.

A therapist is treating a new patient in an outpatient facility. The patient has recently been diagnosed with type I insulin-dependent diabetes mellitus. The patient asks the therapist the differences between type I insulin-dependent diabetes mellitus and type II non–insulin-dependent diabetes mellitus. Which of the following statements is true?

A. There is usually some insulin present in the blood in type I and none in type II.
B. Ketoacidosis is a symptom of type II.
C. The age of diagnosis with type I is usually younger than the age of diagnosis with type II.
D. Both conditions can be managed with a strict diet, only without taking insulin.

Question 271.

At a team meeting, the respiratory therapist informs the rest of the team that the patient, just admitted to the subacute floor, experienced breathing difficulty in the acute care department. The respiratory therapist describes the breathing problem as a pause before exhaling after a full inspiration. Which of the following is the therapist describing?

A. Apnea
B. Orthopnea
C. Eupnea
D. Apneusis

Question 272.

A therapist is asked to evaluate a patient in the intensive care unit. The patient is comatose but breathing independently. During the assessment of range of motion in the right upper extremity, the therapist notices that the patient is breathing unusually. The pattern is an increase in breathing rate and depth followed by brief pauses in breathing. The therapist should notify the appropriate personnel that the patient is exhibiting which of the following patterns?

A. Biot's
B. Cheyne-Stokes
C. Kussmaul's
D. Paroxysmal nocturnal dyspnea

Question 273.

A patient presents to therapy with poor motor control of the lower extremities. The therapist determines that to work efficiently toward the goal of returning the patient to his prior level of ambulation, he must work in the following order regarding stages of control:

A. Mobility, controlled mobility, stability, skill
B. Stability, controlled stability, mobility, skill
C. Skill, controlled stability, controlled mobility
D. Mobility, stability, controlled mobility, skill

Question 274.

A physical therapist is ordered to evaluate a patient in the intensive care unit who recently suffered a stroke. The evaluation reveals the following signs and symptoms: contralateral hemiplegia (upper extremity involvement greater than lower extremities), homonymous hemianopsia, aphasia (due to the dominant hemishpere being involved), and contralateral loss of sensation in the upper extremities. Which of the following arteries is the most likely location of the lesion?

A. Middle cerebral artery
B. Anterior cerebral artery
C. Carotid internal artery
D. Posterior cerebral artery

Question 275.

A physical therapist is treating a patient with significant burns over the limbs and upper trunk. Which of the following statements is false about some of the changes initially experienced after the burn?

A. This patient initially experienced an increase in the number of white blood cells
B. This patient initially experienced an increase in the number of red blood cells
C. This patient initially experienced an increase in the number of free fatty acids
D. This patient initially experienced a decrease in fibrinogen

Question 276.

Each of the following choices consists of a list of two summaries of some of the principles in the code of ethics of the American Physical Therapy Association. Which of the answers below is a false summary?

A. (1) Obey regulations governing physical therapists, and (2) maintain high standards when providing therapy.
B. (1) Respect the rights of patients, and (2) inform people appropriately of the services provided.
C. (1) Maintain high standards when providing therapy, and (2) provide services for the length of time ordered.
D. (1) Assist the public when there are public health needs, and (2) accept fair monetary compensation for services.

Question 277.

A physical therapist is evaluating a patient with muscular dystrophy. The patient seems to "waddle" when she walks. She rolls the right hip forward when advancing the right lower extremity and the left hip forward when advancing the left lower extremity. Which of the following gait patterns is the patient demonstrating?

A. Gluteus maximus gait
B. Dystrophic gait
C. Arthrogenic gait
D. Antalgic

Question 278.

Which of the following statements is not a common physiologic change of aging?

A. Blood pressure taken at rest and during exercise increases
B. Maximal oxygen uptake decreases
C. Residual volume decreases
D. Bone mass decreases

Question 279.

A physical therapist is speaking to a group of pregnant women about maintaining fitness level during pregnancy. Which of the following statements contain incorrect information?

A. Perform regular exercise routines at least three times per week
B. Perform at least fifteen minutes per day of abdominal exercises in supine position, during the second and third trimesters
C. Increase caloric intake by 300 per day
D. Exercise decreases constipation during pregnancy

Question 280.

A physical therapist is ordered to provide gait training to a 78-year-old man who received a right cemented total knee replacement 24 hours earlier. The patient also had a traumatic amputation of the left upper extremity 3 inches above the elbow 40 years ago. If the patient lives at home alone, which of the following is an appropriate assistive device?

A. Rolling walker
B. Standard walker
C. Hemi-walker
D. Wheelchair for 2 weeks

Question 281.

A 48-year-old woman is being evaluated by a physical therapist. Her diagnosis is right rotator cuff tendinitis. She reports right shoulder weakness and pain for the past 2 months. The patient describes "pins and needles" over the lateral right shoulder and upper extremity, extending into the thumb. She also reports no causative trauma. Manual muscle testing reveals in the right upper extremity: flexion = 4/5, extension = 3+/5, abduction = 3+/5, adduction = 4/5, internal rotation = 3+/5, and external rotation = 3+/5. Manual muscle testing reveals in the left upper extremity: flexion = 4+/5, extension = 5/5, abduction = 5/5, adduction = 4+/5, internal rotation = 4+/5, and external rotation = 4+/5. Active and passive shoulder range of motion is within normal limits and equal bilaterally. All thoracic outlet tests are negative. All shoulder special tests are negative. Which of the following steps would most likely assess the source of the patient's problems?

A. Elbow strength and range of motion testing
B. Grip strength testing
C. Cervical spine testing
D. Scapular muscle strength testing

Question 282.

A 23-year-old woman arrives at an outpatient physical therapy clinic with a prescription to evaluate and treat the right hand. One week earlier the patient underwent surgical repair of the flexor tendons of the right hand at zone 2. She also had her cast removed at the physician's office a few minutes before coming to physical therapy. What is the best course of treatment for this patient?

A. Ultrasound to decrease scarring
B. Gentle grip strengthening with putty
C. Splinting the distal interphalangeal joint and proximal interphalangeal joints at neutral
D. Splinting with the use of rubber bands to passively flex the fingers

Question 283.

A physical therapist is performing an isokinetic test on a 16-year-old boy's shoulder. This particular test compares the right shoulder with the left shoulder. The patient's father asks the physical therapist, "What is the purpose of this test?" How should the therapist respond?

A. "This isokinetic test will show changes in concentric and eccentric strength"
B. "This test will show strength differences between the injured arm and the non-injured arm"
C. "This test shows differences in external rotation strength at specific ranges in the arc of motion"
D. "This test will provide muscular torque data which will help us to determine when to discontinue therapy"

Question 284.

A physical therapist in the rehabilitation unit is ordered to evaluate and treat a 3-year-old girl with cerebral palsy. The patient's supportive family is present during the evaluation. When should the physical therapist explain the treatment plan and possible functional outcomes to the family?

A. During the evaluation
B. After the evaluation
C. After the first full treatment session
D. After the first rehabilitation team conference meeting

Question 285.

A physical therapist is treating a 65-year-old man with pneumonia. The patient questions the benefits of the flow incentive spirometer left in the room by the respiratory therapist a few minutes ago. Which of the following is an appropriate response to the patient's question?

A. "It gives visual feedback on lung performance"
B. "It helps you maintain current lung volumes"
C. "You need to ask the respiratory therapist this question"
D. A and B are correct responses

Question 286.

A 53-year-old man with chronic obstructive pulmonary disease reports to an outpatient cardiopulmonary rehabilitation facility. Pulmonary testing reveals that forced expiratory volume in 1 second (FEV_1) and vital capacity (VC) are within 60% of predicted values. What is the appropriate exercise prescription?

A. Exercise at 75–80% of the target heart rate 3 times/week
B. Begin exercise with levels of 1.5 METs and increase slowly 3 times/week
C. Exercise at 75–80% of the target heart rate 7 times/week
D. Begin exercise with levels of 1.5 METs and increase slowly 7 times/week

Question 287.

Which of the following are indications for pulmonary suctioning?

A. Unproductive coughs
B. Breathe sounds of wet rales
C. Respiratory distress
D. All of the above

Question 288.

Which of the following exercises does not increase strength of the muscles of forceful inspiration?

A. Active cervical flexion exercises
B. Active genohumeral extension exercises
C. Shoulder shrugs
D. Crunches

Question 289.

A clinical instructor is explaining to his student how a muscle contracts. The instructor describes tthe cycle of cross-bridging. He begins by stating that the first step is that the cross-bridges attach to the thin filament. Which of the following occurs next (in the correct order)?

A. The attachment with the actin filament is lost. The cross-bridge moves into position to attach to the thick filament. Cross-bridge moves, causing the thin filament to move.
B. The cross-bridge moves into position to attach to the thick filament. The attachment with the myosin filament is lost. Cross-bridge moves, causing the thin filament to move.
C. The attachment with the myosin filament is lost. Cross-bridge moves, causing the myosin filament to move. The cross-bridge moves into position to attach to a myosin filament.
D. Cross-bridge moves, causing the actin filament to move. The attachment with the thin filament is lost. The cross-bridge moves into position to attach to an actin filament.

Question 290.

A therapist is evaluating a wound in a patient with the following signs: the right foot has a toe that is gangrenous, the skin on the dorsum of the foot is shiny in appearance, and no calluses are present. The patient has what type of ulcer?

A. Venous insufficiency ulcer
B. Arterial insufficiency ulcer
C. Decubitus ulcer
D. Trophic ulcer

Question 291.

A physical therapist is beginning an evaluation of a 5-year-old boy. The mother indicates that she pulled the child from a seated position by grasping the wrists. The child then experienced immediate pain at the right elbow. The physician's orders are for right elbow range of motion and strengthening. Which of the following is the most likely diagnosis?

A. Radial head fracture
B. Nursemaid's elbow
C. Erb's palsy
D. Ulnar coronoid process fracture

Question 292.

A physician has ordered a specific type of electrical stimulation that utilizes a frequency of 2500 Hz with a base frequency at 50 Hz to achieve fused tetany. What type of electrical stimulation has the physician ordered?

A. Iontophoresis
B. Transcutaneous electrical nerve stimulation
C. Intermittent flow configuration
D. Russian stimulation

Question 293.

A physical therapist who is pregnant has been studying the use of transcutaneous electrical nerve stimulation during labor and birth to decrease pain perception. Which of the following is the most effective technique in this situation?

A. Place the electrodes over the upper abdominals during the first stages of labor and over the lower abdominals during the later stages
B. Place the electrodes over the paraspinals at the L5 level and S1 level throughout labor and delivery
C. Place the electrodes in a V pattern above the pubic region during labor and delivery
D. Place electrodes over the paraspinals at the L1 and S1 level initially during labor, and over the pubic region during the latter stages

Question 294.

A patient with chronic back pain is referred to physical therapy for application of a transcutaneous electrical nerve stimulation unit. The parameters chosen by the therapist are set to provide a noxius stimulus described as an acupuncture type of stimulus. Which of the following lists of parameters produces this type of stimulation?

A. Low intensity, duration of 60 μsec, and a frequency of 50 Hz
B. High intensity, duration of 150 μsec, and a frequency of 100 Hz
C. Low intensity, duration of 150 μsec, and a frequency of 100 Hz
D. High intensity, duration of 150 μsec, and a frequency of 2 Hz

Question 295.

A 65-year-old man presents to physical therapy with complaints of pain due to compression fractures of the C2 and C3 vertebrae. The patient has an unusually large cranium. He describes his condition by stating, "Much of my bone tissue is continually decreasing, then reforming." The patient also indicates that the condition has caused limb deformity. Which of the following diseases does he have?

A. Paget's disease
B. Achondroplastic dwarfism
C. Osteogenesis imperfecta
D. Osteopetrosis

Question 296.

A patient informs his therapist that his problem began 3 months after a bout of the flu. The patient originally experienced tingling in the hands and feet. He also reports progressive weakness to the point that he required a ventilator to breathe. He is now recovering rapidly and is expected to return to a normal functional level in 3 more months. From which of the following conditions is the patient most likely suffering?

A. Parkinson's disease
B. Guillain-Barré syndrome
C. Multiple sclerosis
D. Amyotrophic lateral sclerosis

Question 297.

A therapist is evaluating a patient in the intensive care unit. The therapist notices that the patient is moving his hands and fingers in slow, writhing motions. Which of the following terms best describes this type of movement?

A. Lead-pipe rigidity
B. Ballisms
C. Chorea
D. Athetosis

Question 298.

A therapist is sent to evaluate a patient with a tumor in the mid-thoracic region. In the chart, the therapist notes that the tumor has been staged using the TNM system. With this system, the letters TNM represent which of the following, in the correct order?

A. Tumor type, number of tumors, tumor metastasis
B. Tumor location, lymph node involved, mass size of the tumor
C. Tumor size, lymph node involvement, tumor metastasis
D. Tumor mass, number of lymph nodes, major organs involved

Question 299.

A physician ordered a splint for a patient who should keep the thumb of the involved hand in abduction. A new graduate is treating the patient and is confused about the difference between thumb flexion, extension, abduction, and adduction. Which of the following lists is correct?

A. Extension is performed in a plane parallel to the palm of the hand, and abduction is performed in a plane perpendicular to the palm of the hand
B. Flexion is performed in a plane perpendicular to the palm of the hand, and adduction is performed in a plane parallel to the palm of the hand
C. Extension is performed in a plane perpendicular to the palm of the hand, and adduction is performed in a plane parallel to the palm of the hand
D. In referring to positions of the thumb, flexion and adduction are used synonymously, and extension and abduction are used synonymously

Question 300.

A patient is referred to physical therapy with complaints of sensation loss over the area of the radius of the right upper extremity, extending from the elbow joint distally to the wrist. Therapy sessions are focused on assisting the patient in regaining normal sensation. Which of the following nerves is responsible for sensation in this region?

A. Medial antebrachial cutaneous
B. Lateral antebrachial cutaneous
C. Musculocutaneous
D. Both B and C

Question 301.

A therapist is evaluating a patient who suffered brain injury in a motor vehicle accident. The somatosensory cortex is involved, resulting in deficits in sensation in the right upper and lower extremities. The therapist knows from visualizing the homunculus that at least part of the injury is in one of the following locations:

A. Inferior right hemisphere of the somatosensory cortex
B. Superior right hemisphere of the somatosensory cortex
C. Inferior left hemisphere of the somatosensory cortex
D. Superior left hemisphere of the somatosensory cortex

Question 302.

While obtaining the subjective history, the therapist learns that the patient was recently hospitalized for malfunction of the anterior pituitary gland. Based on this information alone, the therapist knows that there may be problems with the patient's ability to produce which of the following hormones?

A. Adrenocorticotropic hormone, thyroid-stimulating hormone, growth hormone, follicle-stimulating hormone, luteinizing hormone
B. Insulin and glucagon
C. Epinephrine and norepinephrine
D. Cortisol, androgens, and aldosterone

Question 303.

While evaluating a patient who suffered a complete spinal cord lesion, the therapist notes the following strength grades with manual muscle testing: wrist extensors = 3+/5, elbow extensors = 2+/5, and intrinsic muscles of the hand = 0/5. What is the highest possible level of this lesion?

A. C3
B. C4
C. C5
D. C7

Question 304.

A patient arrives at an outpatient clinic with an order from the physician for whirlpool and wound care to a lower extremity wound. The therapist decides to set the temperature in the whirlpool at warm. Which of the following settings in degrees Celsius is appropriate?

A. 27.5° Celsius
B. 35.5° Celsius
C. 49° Celsius
D. 60° Celsius

Question 305.

A supervisor is asked by a hired architect to provide some of the measurements needed to make a new clinic accessible for people who require wheelchairs. Some of the concerns of the architect are the minimal width of the doorways, the steepest slope allowed for the wheelchair ramp at the front entrance, and the minimal height of the bathroom toilet seat. If the supervisor provided measurements based on normal adult size, which of the following lists of measurements would be correct?

A. The minimal doorway width should be 32 inches. The steepest slope allowed is 1:12 (for every 12 feet of horizontal length, the ramp can rise vertically by 1 foot). The minimal toilet seat height is 17 inches.
B. The minimal doorway width should be 32 inches. The steepest slope allowed is 1:14 (for every 14 feet of horizontal length, the ramp can rise vertically by 1 foot). The minimal toilet seat height is 22 inches.
C. The minimal doorway width should be 30 inches. The steepest slope allowed is 1:12 (for every 12 feet of horizontal length, the ramp can rise vertically by 1 foot). The minimal toilet seat height is 24 inches.
D. The minimal doorway width should be 28 inches. The steepest slope allowed is 1:12 (for every 12 feet of horizontal length, the ramp can rise vertically by 1 foot). The minimal toilet seat height is 15 inches.

Question 306.

A physical therapist is scheduled to evaluate the shoulder of a patient with hepatitis B. The therapist notices no open wounds or abrasions and also notices that the patient has good hygiene. The physician has ordered passive range of motion to the right shoulder because of adhesive capsulitis. Which of the following precautions is absolutely necessary to prevent the therapist from being infected?

A. The therapist must wear a gown
B. The therapist must wear a mask
C. The therapist must wear gloves
D. None of the above

Question 307.

A therapist is performing chest physiotherapy on a patient who is coughing up a significant amount of sputum. The therapist later describes the quality of the sputum in his notes as mucoid. This description tells other personnel which of the following?

A. The sputum is thick
B. The sputum has a foul odor
C. The sputum is clear or white in color
D. The patient has a possible bronchopulmonary infection

Question 308.

A therapist is sent to provide passive range of motion to a patient in the intensive care unit. The chart reveals that the patient is suffering from pulmonary edema. The charge nurse informs the therapist that the patient is coughing up a thin, white sputum with a pink tint. Which of the following terms best describes this sputum?

A. Purulent
B. Frothy
C. Mucopurulent
D. Rusty

Question 309.

A therapist is screening a patient complaining of pain at the anterior left shoulder region. The pain is increased when the examiner instructs the patient to position the left arm by his side with the elbow flexed at 90° and to actively supinate the forearm against resistance (provided by the examiner). What test is being performed?

A. Froment's sign
B. Yergason's test
C. Waldron test
D. Wilson test

Question 310.

A physical therapist must have a clear understanding of the normal development of the human body to treat effectively and efficiently. Which of the following principles of treatment is incorrect?

A. Early motor activity is influenced primarily by reflexes
B. Motor control develops from proximal to distal and from head to toe
C. Increasing motor ability is independent of motor learning
D. Early motor activity is influenced by spontaneous activity

Question 311.

A patient with cardiac arrhythmia is referred to physical therapy services for cardiac rehabilitation. The therapist is aware that the heart receives nerve impulses that begin in the sinoatrial node of the heart and then proceed to which of the following:

A. Atrioventricular node, then to the Purkinje fibers, and then to the bundle branches
B. Purkinje fibers, then to the bundle branches, and then to the atrioventricular node
C. Atrioventricular node, then to the bundle branches, and then to the Purkinje fibers
D. Bundle branches, then to the atrioventricular node, and then to the Purkinje fibers

Question 312.

A physical therapist receives an order from the physician to treat a patient using iontophoresis. The order indicates that the purpose of the treatment is to attempt to dissolve a calcium deposit in the area of the Achilles' tendon. When preparing the patient for treatment, the therapist connects the medicated electrode to the negative pole. Which of the following medications is the therapist most likely preparing to administer?

A. Dexamethasone
B. Magnesium sulfate
C. Hydrocortisone
D. Acetic acid

Question 313.

A therapist is assisting a patient in gaining lateral stability of the knee joint. The therapist is using strengthening exercises to strengthen muscle groups that will increase active restraint on the lateral side of the joint. Which of the following offers the least amount of active lateral restraint?

A. Gastrocnemius
B. Popliteus
C. Biceps femoris
D. Iliotibial band

Question 314.

A clinical instructor is explaining to a physical therapy student the function of the screw home mechanism in the knee joint. Part of the therapist's explanation involves teaching the student the movement of the tibia and femur during closed-chain activities. When the knee joint is extended in a closed-chain activity, which of the following statements is true?

A. The femur laterally rotates on the tibia
B. The femur medially rotates on the tibia
C. The tibia laterally rotates on the femur
D. The tibia medially rotates on the femur

Question 315.

A therapist is evaluating a patient with traumatic injury to the left hand. The therapist asks the patient to place the left hand on the examination table with the palm facing upward. The therapist then holds the second, third, and fifth digits in full extension. The patient is then asked to flex the fourth digit. What movement would be expected by a patient with an uninjured hand, and what muscle or muscles is the therapist restricting?

A. The fourth finger would flex at the distal interphalangeal (DIP) joint only, and the muscle being restricted would be the flexor digitorum superficialis
B. The fourth finger would flex at the proximal interphalangeal (PIP) joint only, and the muscle being restricted would be the flexor digitorum profundus
C. The fourth finger would flex at the DIP joint only, and the muscles being restricted would be the lumbricals
D. The fourth finger would flex at the PIP joint only, and the muscles being restricted would be the palmar interosseous

Question 316.

A 67-year-old man with a below-knee amputation presents to an outpatient clinic. His surgical amputation was 3 weeks ago, and his scars are well healed. Which of the following is incorrect information about stump care?

A. Use a light lotion on the stump after bathing each night
B. Continue with use of a shrinker 12 hours per day
C. Wash the stump with mild soap and water
D. Scar massage techniques

Question 317.

A patient is in prone position with his head rotated to the left side. The left upper extremity is placed at his side and fully internally rotated. The left shoulder is then shrugged toward the chin. The therapist then grasps the midshaft of the patient's left forearm. The patient is then instructed to "try to reach your feet using just your left arm." This movement is resisted by the therapist. This test is assessing the strength of what muscle?

A. Upper trapezius
B. Posterior deltoid
C. Latissimus dorsi
D. Triceps brachii

Question 318.

Which of the following is a false statement about below-knee amputations?

A. Gel socket inserts should be left in the prosthesis overnight
B. The therapist should puncture any blisters that appear on the stump
C. Areas of skin irritation on the stump can be covered with a dressing, then a nylon sock before donning the prosthesis
D. When not in use the prosthesis should be lain on the floor

Question 319.

A therapist is assisting a patient with pre-gait activities who has been fitted with a hip disarticulation prosthesis. To ambulate with the most correct gait pattern, what must be mastered first?

A. Forward weight shift on to the prosthesis
B. Swing-through of the prosthesis
C. Maintain stability while in single limb support on the prosthesis
D. Posterior pelvic tilt to advance the prosthesis

Question 320.

A 63-year-old woman presents to physical therapy with a diagnosis of herpes zoster. The physician informs the physical therapist that the L5 dorsal root is involved and that a transcutaneous electrical neuromuscular stimulation (TENS) unit should be used to help control the pain. Where should the TENS unit electrodes be placed?

A. Posterior thigh
B. Lateral hip/greater trochanter area
C. Anterior thigh
D. Anterior lateral tibia

Question 321.

A physical therapist is teaching a class in geriatric fitness/strengthening at a local gym. Which of the following is not a general guideline for exercise prescription in this patient population?

A. To increase exercise intensity, increase treadmill speed rather than the grade
B. Start at a low intensity (2–3 METs)
C. Use machines for strength training rather than free weights
D. Set weight resistance so that the patient can perform more than 8 repetitions before fatigue

Question 322.

A 63-year-old man presents to an outpatient physical therapy clinic with a diagnosis of sciatica. The MRI report is negative for lumbar disc involvement. During the evaluation the physical therapist cannot reproduce the symptoms of radiculopathy with any test. Lower extremity strength is equal bilaterally and is not weak in any particular pattern. The patient informs the therapist that the pain is bilateral, located in the gastrocnemius area, and increases with prolonged ambulation. The pain stops soon after resting in a seated position. What is the most likely source of this patient's pain?

A. Impingement of the L5 dorsal root
B. Multiple sclerosis
C. Compartment syndrome
D. Intermittent claudication

Question 323.

Which of the following is widely considered the most accurate body composition assessment?

A. Hydrostatic weighing
B. Electrical impedance
C. Anthropometric measurement
D. None of the above

Question 324.

A physical therapist is evaluating a 5-day old infant with cerebral palsy. The infant has an abnormal amount of extensor tone. Which of the following is correct positioning advice for the family and nursing staff?

A. Keep the infant in supine position
B. Keep the infant in prone position
C. Keep the infant in sidelying position
D. B and C are correct

Question 325.

A 76-year-old woman received a cemented right total hip arthroplasty (THA) 24 hours ago. The surgeon documented that he used a posterolateral incision. Which of the following suggestions is inappropriate for the next 24 hours?

A. Avoid hip flexion above 30°
B. Avoid hip adduction past midline
C. Avoid any internal rotation
D. Avoid abduction past 15°

Question 326.

A physical therapist is treating a 76-year-old woman with left lower extremity hypotonia secondary to a recent stroke. Which of the following is an incorrect method to normalize tone?

A. Rapid irregular movements
B. Approximation
C. Prolonged stretch
D. Tactile cues

Question 327.

An 81-year-old woman with right-side hemiparesis due to stroke is being treated by a physical therapist through home health services. The therapist is attempting to increase the functional reach of the right upper extremity. The patient currently has 120° of active flexion. The therapist decides to use trunk mobility/stability facilitation techniques to help achieve the patient's functional goals. Which of the following skills need to be mastered by the patient to attain the ability to reach 2 feet in front of her wheelchair and 2 feet to the right of midline at 125° of shoulder flexion with the right upper extremity?

A. Weight shifting to the left buttock and right-side trunk elongation
B. Weight shifting to the left buttock and left-side trunk elongation
C. Weight shifting to the right buttock and right-side trunk elongation
D. Weight shifting to the right buttock and left-side trunk elongation

Question 328.

Which of the following statements about developmental motor control is incorrect?

A. Isotonic control develops before isometric control
B. Gross motor control develops prior to fine motor control
C. Eccentric movement develops prior to concentric movement
D. Trunk control develops prior to distal extremity control

Question 329.

A therapist is attempting to open the spastic and flexed hand of a patient who has suffered a recent stroke. Which of the following does not inhibit hand opening?

A. Avoid touching the interossei
B. Apply direct pressure to the thenar eminence
C. Hyperextend the metacarpophalangeal joint
D. A and B

Question 330.

A 65-year-old man is scheduled to begin a wellness program. He has no cardiovascular disease, major systemic illness, or musculoskeletal abnormality. However, he is deconditioned because of an extremely sedentary lifestyle. Resting heart rate is 90 beats/minute, and resting blood pressure is 145/92 mmHg. Which of the choices below describes the most correct intensity, frequency, and duration at which the patient should begin exercise?

A. 75% VO_2 max; 30 minutes/day; 3 days/week
B. 40% VO_2 max; 30 minutes/day; 5 days/week
C. 40% VO_2 max; 10 minutes twice daily; 5 days/week
D. 75% VO_2 max; 10 minutes twice daily; 3 days/week

Question 331.

Which of the following is the normal end-feel perceived by an examiner assessing wrist flexion?

A. Bone to bone
B. Soft tissue approximation
C. Tissue stretch
D. Empty

Question 332.

A physical therapist is beginning an evaluation of a patient with a diagnosis of "knee strain." Range of motion limitation does not follow the normal capsular pattern of the knee. Which of the following are possible causes of the restriction in range of motion?

A. Ligamentous adhesions
B. Internal derangement
C. Extra-articular lesions
D. All of the above

Question 333.

A child presents to physical therapy with a diagnosis of right Sever's disease. What joint should be the focus of the therapist's evaluation?

A. Right knee joint
B. Right hip joint
C. Right wrist joint
D. Right ankle joint

Question 334.

A physical therapist is reviewing the chart of a 24-year-old woman with a diagnosis of L2 incomplete paraplegia. The physician noted that the left quadricep tendon reflex is 2+. What does this information relay to the therapist?

A. No active quadricep tendon reflex
B. Slight quadricep contraction with reflex testing
C. Normal quadricep tendon reflex
D. Exaggerated quadricep tendon reflex

Question 335.

A physical therapist performs the following test during an evaluation: With the patient lying in supine position, the therapist traces a diamond shape around the patient's umbilicus with a sharp object. What reflex is being assessed, and what is the significance if the patient's umbilicus does not move in response to the stimulus provided by the therapist?

A. Cremaster reflex; suggests upper motor neuron involvement
B. Superficial abdominal reflex; suggests upper motor neuron involvement
C. Cremaster reflex; suggests lower motor neuron involvement
D. Superficial abdominal reflex; suggests lower motor neuron involvement

Question 336.

A 29-year-old woman who is 8 months pregnant presents to an outpatient clinic with complaints of "pain and tingling" over the lateral thigh. She also indicates no traumatic injury. The symptoms increase after she has been sitting for 30 minutes or longer, and the overall intensity of the symptoms has been increasing over the past 2 weeks. The therapist notes that repeated active lumbar flexion does not increase pain, and the patient's lumbar range of motion is normal for a pregnant woman. There is also no motor weakness in the hip or pelvis, and the sacroiliac joint is not abnormally rotated. What is the most probable diagnosis?

A. L3 disc dysfunction
B. Spondylolisthesis
C. L4 disc dysfunction
D. Meralgia paresthetica

Question 337.

The therapist is evaluating a 38-year-old man who complains of right sacroiliac joint pain. The therapist decides to assess leg length discrepancy in supine vs. sitting position. When the patient is in supine position, leg lengths are equal; however, when the patient rises to the sitting position, the right lower extremity appears 2 cm shorter. Which of the following should be a part of the treatment plan?

A. Right posterior SI mobilization
B. Right anterior SI mobilization
C. Left posterior SI mobilization
D. Left anterior SI mobilization

Question 338.

In taping an athlete's ankle prophylactically before a football game, in what position should the ankle be slightly positioned before taping to provide the most protection against an ankle sprain?

A. Inversion, dorsiflexion, abduction
B. Eversion, plantarflexion, adduction
C. Eversion, dorsiflexion, abduction
D. Inversion, plantarflexion, adduction

Question 339.

Which of the following is inappropriate for a physical therapist to include in the treatment plan of an infant with a gestational age of 27 weeks and Down's syndrome?

A. Bottle feeding
B. Encourage sidelying position
C. Tactile stimulation with the entire hand rather that the fingertips of the examiner
D. Prone positioning

Question 340.

Which of the following sources of stimulation is least effective in obtaining functional goals when treating an infant with decreased muscular tone?

A. Vestibular
B. Weight-bearing
C. Cutaneous
D. Vibratory

Question 341.

Which of the following is the most important goal in treating pediatric patients with postural reaction deficits?

A. Age-appropriate responses
B. Automatic responses
C. Conscious responses
D. Lower extremity control before upper extremity control

Question 342.

Which of the following statements best describes lower extremity positioning in standing during the first 2 years of life of a child with no dysfunction?

A. Femoral anteversion, femoral external rotation, foot pronation
B. Femoral anteversion, femoral internal rotation, foot supination
C. Femoral retroversion, femoral external rotation, foot pronation
D. Femoral retroversion, femoral internal rotation, foot supination

Question 343.

A 10-year-old boy presents to outpatient physical therapy with complaints of diffuse pain in the right hip, thigh, and knee joint. The patient was involved in a motor vehicle accident 3 weeks ago. He is also obese and has significant atrophy in the right quadricep. The right lower extremity is held by the patient in the position of flexion, abduction, and lateral rotation. Which of the following is most likely the source of the patient's signs and symptoms?

A. Greater trochanteric bursitis
B. Avascular necrosis
C. Slipped femoral capital epiphysis
D. Septic arthritis

Question 344.

A physical therapist is treating a 35-year-old man with traumatic injury to the right hand. The patient has several surgical scars from a tendon repair performed 6 weeks ago. What is the appropriate type of masssage for the patient's scars?

A. Transverse and longitudinal
B. Circular and longitudinal
C. Transverse and circular
D. Massage is contraindicated after a tendon repair

Question 345.

Which of the following statements is true in comparing infants with Down's syndrome to infants with no known abnormalities?

A. Motor milestones are reached at the same time with both groups
B. Postural reactions are developed in the same time frame with both groups
C. Postural reactions and motor milestones are developed slower in patients who have Down's syndrome, but with the same association as with normal infants
D. Postural reactions and motor milestones are not developed with the same association with patients who have Down's syndrome as with normal infants

Question 346.

A high-school athlete is considering whether to have an anterior cruciate ligament reconstruction. The therapist explains the importance of this ligament, especially in a person that is young and athletic. Which of the statements below is correct in describing part of the function of the anterior cruciate ligament?

A. The anterior cruciate ligament prevents excessive posterior roll of the femoral condyles during flexion of the femur at the knee joint
B. The anterior cruciate ligament prevents excessive anterior roll of the femoral condyles during flexion of the femur at the knee joint
C. The anterior cruciate ligament prevents excessive posterior roll of the femoral condyles during extension of the femur at the knee joint
D. The anterior cruciate ligament prevents excessive anterior roll of the femoral condyles during extension of the femur at the knee joint

Question 347.

A therapist is evaluating a patient in the intensive care unit. While performing a chart review, the therapist discovers that the patient was seriously injured in a fall from a 3-story building. The therapist determines from the physician's evaluation that of the many injuries the patient has sustained, a rupture of two ligaments extends from the side of the dens to the medial side of the occipital condyle. Which of the following was injured?

A. Ligamentum nuchae
B. Tectorial membrane
C. Posterior atlanto-occipital ligament
D. Alar ligament

Question 348.

A physical therapist is treating an 81-year-old man with Parkinson's disease. The patient has been ambulating with a cane. He was referred to physical therapy because of a fall at home. The family reports a decrease in gait ability during the past several months. The therapist decides to begin gait training with a rolling walker. Which of the following is incorrect for the treatment of this patient?

A. Strengthening of the hip flexors, and stretching of the gluteals
B. Slow, rhythmical rocking techniques
C. Biofeedback during ambulation
D. Prolonged passive stretching of the gastrocnemius muscle group bilaterally

Question 349.

A patient is in an outpatient facility because of an injury sustained to the right knee joint. Only the structures within the synovial cavity were compromised during the injury. Knowing this information only, the therapist is not concerned with injury to which of the following structures?

A. Patellofemoral joint
B. Anterior cruciate ligament
C. Medial meniscus
D. Femoral condyles

Question 350.

A 14-year-old girl presents to an outpatient physical therapy clinic with complaints of anterior knee pain for 2 weeks. The patient notes no particular incident of onset. She indicates that pain increases when she attempts to ascend and descend stairs and with squatting to 130° of knee flexion. The evaluation shows limited quadricep strength on the involved side at 4/5 with manual muscle testing and normal hamstring strength. All meniscus and ligament tests are negative. Given the above information, what is the most likely cause of the signs and symptoms?

A. Lateral glide of the patella
B. Medial tilt of the patella
C. Baker's cyst
D. Anterior cruciate ligament tear

Question 351.

Which of the following is the best treatment plan for the above patient?

A. Patellofemoral taping, open chain quadricep strengthening at 90–45° of flexion, closed chain quadricep strengthening at 45–0° of flexion
B. Patellofemoral taping, open chain quadricep strengthening at 45–0° of flexion, closed chain quadricep strengthening at 90–45° of flexion
C. Hamstring strengthening, terminal knee extension exercises, and ice
D. B and C

Question 352.

A patient with decreased function of the gluteus minimus is referred to physical therapy for gait training. During the evaluation, the therapist places the patient in prone position and instructs the patient to extend the hip. Knowing that the gluteus minimus is extremely weak, which of the following is most likely to happen?

A. The patient will abduct the hip more than usual when attempting to perform hip extension
B. The patient will externally rotate the hip excessively when attempting to perform hip extension
C. The patient will excessively flex the knee when attempting to perform hip extension
D. The patient will not have difficulty performing straight hip extension

Question 353.

A patient is placed in supine position with the knee in 90° of flexion. The foot is stabilized by the therapist's body on the examination table. The therapist then wraps his fingers around the proximal tibia so that the thumbs are resting along the anteromedial and the anterolateral margins. The therapist then applies a force to pull the tibia forward. What special test is being performed?

A. Pivot shift
B. Lachman's test
C. Anterior drawer
D. Posterior drawer

Question 354.

A therapist is evaluating a patient who complains of frequent foot, ankle, and knee pain. The therapist asks the patient to assume a standing position with the knees slightly flexed. The therapist then demonstrates active bilateral foot pronation to the patient. When asked to perform this task, the patient has difficulty. Which of the following limitations is a possible cause of the patient's difficulty in performing this task?

A. Restriction limiting plantar flexion and lateral rotation of the talus
B. Restriction limiting dorsiflexion and medial rotation of the talus
C. Restriction limiting eversion of the calcaneus and medial rotation of the talus
D. B and C are correct

Question 355.

Of the following, which is the earliest period after surgery that an 18-year-old boy who received an uncomplicated partial meniscectomy of the right knee can perform functional testing, such as a one-leg hop test, for distance?

A. 1 week after surgery
B. 2 weeks after surgery
C. 6 weeks after surgery
D. 12 weeks after surgery

Question 356.

A patient is being evaluated by a physical therapist because of bilateral knee pain. The therapist is attempting to rule out ankle or foot dysfunction as the source of the pain. Which of the following observations is not true in evaluating a patient without foot or ankle problems in the standing position?

A. The talus is situated somewhat medially to the midline of the foot
B. In quiet standing the muscles surrounding the ankle joint remain silent
C. The first and second metatarsal heads bear more weight than the fourth and fifth metatarsal heads
D. The talus transmits weight to the rest of the bones of the foot

Question 357.

A physical therapist is evaluating of a female distance runner who complains of intermittent medial ankle pain. In static standing, the therapist palpates excessive lateral deviation of the head of the talus. From this information, in what position is the subtalar joint during palpation?

A. Supination
B. Pronation
C. Neutral
D. Unable to determine from the information given

Question 358.

A patient presents to therapy with an ankle injury. The therapist has determined that the injury is at the junction of the distal tibia and fibula. Which of the following functions most in preventing excessive external rotation and posterior displacement of the fibula?

A. Anterior inferior tibiofibular ligament
B. Posterior inferior tibiofibular ligament
C. Interosseous membrane
D. None of the above

Question 359.

A physical therapist is asked to evaluate a 37-year-old man with right-side sciatica. The therapist performs a passive straight-leg raise test of the right lower extremity with the knee and ankle in neutral position. In performing this test on a patient with an L5 disc protrusion, what is the lowest degree at which the therapist would expect to reproduce the patient's symptoms?

A. At 0° of hip flexion
B. At 35° of hip flexion
C. At 70° of hip flexion
D. At 90° of hip flexion

Question 360.

A patient is being treated in an outpatient facility after receiving a meniscus repair to the right knee 1 week ago. The patient has full passive extension of the involved knee but lacks 4° of full extension when performing a straight leg raise. The patient's active flexion is 110° and passive flexion is 119°. What is a common term used to describe the patient's most significant range of motion deficit? What is a possible source of this problem?

A. Flexion contracture—quadricep atrophy
B. Extension lag—joint effusion
C. Flexion lag—weak quadriceps
D. Extension contracture—tight hamstrings

Question 361.

A 17-year-old athlete has just received a posterior cruciate ligament reconstruction. The therapist is attempting to explain some of the characteristics of the posterior cruciate ligament. Which of the following is incorrect information?

A. The posterior cruciate ligament prevents posterior translation of the tibia on the femur
B. Posterior bands of the posterior cruciate ligament are their tightest in full knee extension
C. The posterior cruciate ligament is attached to the lateral meniscus and not to the medial meniscus
D. The posterior cruciate ligament helps with medial rotation of the tibia during full knee extension with open chain activities

Question 362.

A physical therapist is evaluating a patient who complains of posterior ankle pain. The patient is positioned prone with the feet extended over the edge of the mat. The therapist squeezes the involved gastrocnemius over the middle third of the muscle belly. What test is the therapist performing? What indicates a positive test?

A. Thompson's test—plantar flexion of the ankle
B. Homan's test—plantar flexion of the ankle
C. Thompson's test—no ankle movement
D. Homan's test—no ankle movement

Question 363.

A patient who has suffered a recent stroke is being treated by a physical therapist. The patient exhibits increased extensor tone in the supine position along with an exaggerated symmetric tonic labyrinthine reflex (STLR). What is the best position to initiate flexion movements of the lower extremity?

A. Prone position
B. Sidelying position
C. Supine position
D. A and B

Question 364.

A physical therapist is attempting to increase a patient's functional mobility in a seated position. To treat the patient most effectively and efficiently, the following should be performed in what order?

1 • Weight shifting of the pelvis
2 • Isometric contractions of the lower extremity
3 • Trunk range of motion exercises
4 • Isotonic resistance to the quadriceps

A. 1,2,3,4
B. 2,3,1,4
C. 4,3,2,1
D. 3,2,1,4

Question 365.

A 14-year-old girl placed excessive valgus stress to the right elbow during a fall from a bicycle. Her forearm was in supination at the moment the valgus stress was applied. Which of the following is most likely involved in this type of injury?

A. Ulnar nerve
B. Extensor carpi radialus
C. Brachioradialis
D. Annular ligament

Question 366.

Which tendon is most commonly involved with lateral epicondylitis?

A. Extensor carpi radialis longus
B. Extensor carpi radialis brevis
C. Brachioradialis
D. Extensor digitorum

Question 367.

A physical therapist is speaking to a group of avid tennis players. The group asks how to prevent tennis elbow (lateral epicondylitis). Which of the following is incorrect information?

A. Primarily use the wrist and elbow extensors during a backhand stroke
B. Begin the backhand stroke in shoulder adduction and internal rotation
C. Use a racket that has a large grip
D. Use a light racket

Question 368.

Which of the following is not part of the triangular fibrocartilage complex of the wrist?

A. Dorsal radioulnar ligament
B. Ulnar collateral ligament
C. Radial collateral ligament
D. Ulnar articular cartilage

Question 369.

Which of the following is the correct method to test for interossei muscular tightness of the hand?

A. Passively flex the proximal interphalangeal (PIP) joints with the metaphalangeal (MP) joints in extension, then passively flex the PIP joints with the MP joints in flexion. Record the difference in PIP joint passive flexion.
B. Passively extend the PIP joints with the MP joints in extension, then passively extend the PIP joints with the MP joints in flexion. Record the difference in PIP joint passive flexion.
C. Passively flex the PIP joints with the MP joints in extension, then passively extend the PIP joints with the MP joints in flexion. Record the difference in PIP joint passive flexion.
D. Passively extend the PIP joints with the MP joints in extension, then passively flex the PIP joints with the MP joints in flexion. Record the difference in PIP joint passive flexion.

Question 370.

A therapist is beginning an evaluation of a 34-year-old woman with a diagnosis of carpal tunnel syndrome. Part of the evaluation consists of grip strength testing. To accurately test strength of the flexor digitorum profundus, where should the grip dynamometer's adjustable handle be placed?

A. 1 inch from the dynamometer's nonadjustable handle
B. 3 inches from the dynamometer's nonadjustable handle
C. 1.5 inches from the dynamometer's nonadjustable handle
D. All of the above are equally effective

Question 371.

A patient who has suffered a zone 2 rupture of the extensor tendon of the 3rd digit presents to physical therapy. This patient had a surgical fixation of the avulsed tendon. During the period of immobilization, which of the following deformities is most likely to develop?

A. Boutonniére deformity.
B. Claw hand.
C. Swan neck deformity.
D. Dupuytren's contracture.

Question 372.

Which of the following muscle tendons most commonly sublux in patient's who suffer from rheumatoid arthritis?

A. Flexor digitorum profundus
B. Extensor carpi ulnaris
C. Extensor carpi radialis longus
D. Flexor pollicis longus

Question 373.

A physical therapist is fabricating a splint for a patient who received four metacarpophalangeal joint replacements. The surgical joint replacement was necessary because severe rheumatoid arthritis. Which of the following is the correct placement of the metacarpophalangeal joints in the splint?

A. Full flexion and slight radial pull
B. Full flexion and slight ulnar pull
C. Full extension and slight radial pull
D. Full extension and slight ulnar pull

Question 374.

A patient presents to an outpatient clinic with an order to evaluate and treat the right forearm and wrist secondary to nerve compression. The patient has the following signs and symptoms: pain with manual muscle testing of pronation; decreased strength of the flexor pollicis longus and pronator quadratus; and pain with palpation of the pronator teres. What nerve is most likely compromised? What is the most likely area of compression?

A. Median nerve—carpal tunnel
B. Ulnar nerve—Guyon's canal
C. Ulnar nerve—pronator quadratus
D. Median nerve—pronator teres

Question 375.

A therapist is ordered to fabricate a splint for a 2-month-old infant with congenital hip dislocation. In what position should the hip be placed while in the splint?

A. Flexion and adduction
B. Extension and adduction
C. Extension and abduction
D. Flexion and abduction

Question 376.

A 30-year-old woman who had a full-term infant 4 weeks ago presents to physical therapy with diastasis recti. The separation was measured by the physician and found to be 3 cm. Which of the following exercises is most appropriate to minimize the separation?

A. Sit-ups while using the upper extremities to bring the rectus abdominis to midline
B. Bridges while using the upper extremities to bring the rectus abdominis to midline
C. Dynamic lumbar stabilization exercises in quadraped position
D. Gentle head lifts in supine position while using the upper extremities to bring the rectus abdominis to midline

Question 377.

A patient presents to outpatient physical therapy with tarsal tunnel syndrome. What nerve is involved? Where should the therapist concentrate treatment?

A. Superficial peroneal nerve—inferior to the medial malleolus
B. Posterior tibial nerve—inferior to the medial malleolus
C. Superficial peroneal nerve—inferior to the lateral malleolus
D. Posterior tibial nerve—inferior to the lateral malleolus

Question 378.

A physical therapist is discharging a 32-year-old man from outpatient physical therapy. The patient received therapy for a traumatic ankle injury that occurred several months prior. The surgery performed on the patient's ankle required placement of plates and screws, which resulted in a permanent range of motion deficit of 10° of active and passive dorsiflexion. Strength in the ankle is 5/5 with manual muscle testing. Of the following, which is the highest functional outcome that the patient can expect?

A. Independent ambulation with no gait deviations
B. Ambulation with a cane with minimal gait deviations
C. Running with no gait deviations
D. Ascend or descend stairs with no gait deviations

Question 379.

A physical therapist is performing passive range of motion on the shoulder of a 43-year-old woman who received a rotator cuff repair 5 weeks ago. During passive range of motion, the therapist notes a capsular end feel at 95° of shoulder flexion. What should the therapist do?

A. Continue with passive range of motion
B. Begin joint mobilization
C. Schedule the patient an appointment with the physician immediately
D. A and B

Question 380.

A physical therapist is treating a 40-year-old business executive who lives a sedentary lifestyle. The patient tires quickly and complains of quadriceps fatigue and "burning" after 2 minutes on the stair stepper. The therapist explains to the patient that the "burning" is probably due to lactic acid build-up in the muscles. Which of the following statements is incorrect?

A. Lactic acid build-up is due to the aerobic system not keeping up with the energy demands of the muscles
B. Lactic acid builds up more quickly in an unconditioned person than in a conditioned person exercising at the same intensity level
C. A small amount of lactic acid is produced at low to moderate intensity levels of exercise
D. Only the anaerobic system is active during rest

Question 381.

A physical therapist is attempting to explain the importance of slow stretching to an athlete training to compete in a marathon. The therapist explains that quick stretching often causes the muscle to _____, which is a response initiated by the _____ , which are located in the muscle fibers. Fill in the blanks.

A. Relax—Golgi tendon organs
B. Contract—Golgi tendon organs
C. Relax—muscle spindles
D. Contract—muscle spindles

Question 382.

In which of the following situations should the therapist be most concerned about the complications resulting from grade IV joint mobilization techniques?

A. A 37-year-old man with a Colles' fracture suffered 10 weeks ago
B. A 23-year-old woman with a boxer's fracture suffered 10 weeks ago
C. A 34-year-old man with a scaphoid fracture suffered 12 weeks ago
D. A 53-year-man with a Bennett's fracture suffered 12 weeks ago

Question 383.

A physical therapist is evaluating a 17-year-old distance runner with complaints of lateral knee pain. During the evaluation, the therapist performs the following test: The patient is placed in supine position with the hip flexed to 45° and the knee to 90°. The therapist then places firm pressure over the lateral femoral epicondyle and extends the patient's knee. Pain is felt by the patient at the point of palpation when her knee is 30° from full knee extension. The positive result of this test suggests which of the following structures as the source of pain?

A. Iliotibial band
B. Biceps femoris
C. Quadriceps
D. Lateral collateral ligament

Question 384.

When ambulating on uneven terrain, how should the subtalar joint be positioned to allow forefoot rotational compensation?

A. Pronation
B. Supination
C. Neutral position
D. The position of the subtalar joint does not influence forefoot compensation

Question 385.

Which of the following is an inappropriate exercise for a patient who received an anterior cruciate ligament reconstruction with a patella tendon autograft 2 weeks ago?

A. Lateral step-ups
B. Heel slides
C. Stationary bike
D. Pool walking

Question 386.

A physical therapist is speaking to a group of receptionists about correct posture. Which of the following is incorrect information?

A. Position computer monitors at eye level
B. Position seats so that the feet are flat on the floor while sitting
C. Position keyboards so that the wrists are in approximately 20° of extension
D. Take frequent stretching breaks

Question 387.

A physical therapist is treating an automobile mechanic. The patient asks for tips on preventing upper extremity repetitive motion injuries. Which of the following is incorrect advice?

A. Use your entire hand rather than just the fingers when holding an object
B. Position tasks so that they are performed below shoulder height
C. Use tools with small straight handles when possible
D. When performing a forceful task, keep the materials slightly lower than the elbow

Question 388.

A physical therapist is treating a 17-year-old boy who suffered a traumatic brain injury. The patient has been in stage IV of the Rancho Los Amigos Cognitive Functioning Scale for 1 week. Which of the following is an inappropriate treatment approach?

A. Start treatment at the same time each day
B. Teach wheelchair safety techniques
C. Change treatment if the patient shows a decrease in interest
D. Give the patient many different exercises options

Question 389.

A 43-year-old man with right biceps brachii rupture presents to physical therapy after a surgical repair. According to the surgeon, the rupture was at the musculotendinous junction. Which of the following has most likely been compromised?

A. Meissner's corpuscles
B. Merkel's disks
C. Ruffini endings
D. Golgi tendon organs

Question 390.

A patient presents to physical therapy with a long-standing diagnosis of bilateral pes planus. The therapist has given the patient custom-fit orthotics. After using the orthotics for 1 week, the patient complains of pain along the first metatarsal. The therapist decides to use joint mobilization techniques to decrease the patient's pain. In which direction should the therapist mobilize the first metatarsal?

A. Inferiorly
B. Superiorly
C. Laterally
D. A and C

Question 391.

A physical therapist begins gait training for a patient with bilateral knee flexion contractures at 30° at a long-term care facility. The therapist knows that the patient will have a forward trunk lean during gait because:

A. The patient's line of gravity is anterior to the hip
B. The patient's line of gravity is anterior to the knee
C. The patient's line of gravity is anterior to the ankle
D. A and C

Question 392.

A therapist is scheduled to evaluate a patient with a chronic condition of "hammer toes." Where should the therapist expect to find callus formation?

A. The distal tips of the toes
B. The superior surface of the interphalangeal joints
C. The metatarsal heads
D. All of the above

Question 393.

What motion takes place at the lumbar spine with right lower extremity single limb support during the gait cycle?

A. Left lateral flexion
B. Right lateral flexion
C. Extension
D. Flexion

Question 394.

An outpatient physical therapist is gait-training a patient recently discharged from the hospital. The inpatient therapist's notes describe a decrease in left stride length due to pain with weight-bearing on the right lower extremity. The outpatient therapist knows that the patient's gait deviation is:

A. An abnormally short distance from the left heel strike and the successive right heel strike
B. An abnormally short amount of time between the left heel strike and the successive right heel strike
C. An abnormally short amount of time in stance phase on the left lower extremity
D. An abnormally short distance between the left heel strike and the successive left heel strike

Question 395.

In the terminal swing phase of gait, what muscles of the foot and ankle are active?

A. Extensor digitorum longus
B. Gastrocnemius
C. Tibialis posterior
D. B and C

Question 396.

A physical therapist is beginning a gait evaluation. During heel strike to foot flat on the right lower extremity, which of the following does not normally occur?

A. The left side of the pelvis initiates movement in the direction of travel
B. The right femur medially rotates
C. The left side of the thorax initiates movement in the direction of travel
D. The right tibia medially rotates

Question 397.

When the knee is at its maximal amount of flexion during the gait cycle, which of the following muscles are active concentrically?

A. Hamstrings
B. Gluteus maximus
C. Gastrocnemius
D. All of the above

Question 398.

When comparing the gait cycle of young adults to the gait cycle of older adults, what would a therapist expect to find?

A. The younger population has a shorter step length
B. The younger population has a shorter stride length
C. The younger population has a shorter period of double support
D. The younger population has a decrease in speed of ambulation

Question 399.

A therapist is treating a patient with a venous insufficiency ulcer over the medial mallelous. The wound is moist and not infected. The involved lower extremity is swollen, and the patient reports no pain around the wound. The physician has ordered wound care 3 times/week. Which of the following is the best treatment?

A. Warm whirlpool
B. Unna boot dressing between therapy sessions
C. Intermittent compression pump
D. B and C

Question 400.

A 68-year-old man is being treated by a physical therapist after a right below-knee amputation. The patient is beginning ambulation with a preparatory prosthesis. In the early stance phase of the involved lower extremity, the therapist notes an increase in knee flexion. Which of the following are possible causes of this gait deviation?

A. The heel is too stiff
B. The foot is set too far anterior in relation to the knee
C. The foot is set in too much plantar flexion
D. All of the above

Answers and Explanations

1. The answer is A.

This deviation is commonly referred to as a lateral heel whip. Excessive internal rotation of the prosthetic knee is one of the causes of this deviation. Excessive external rotation of the knee causes a medial heel whip.

2. The answer is D.

The long toe extensors represent the spinal cord segment L5. The iliopsoas represents L2. The quadriceps are innervated by L3 and the tibialis anterior is innervated by L4.

3. The answer is A.

Verapamil reduces contractility of the heart and increases coronary artery dilation, resulting in decreased cardiac workload and increased blood flow to the heart muscle.

4. The answer is B.

The superior angle of the scapula commonly rests at the same level as vertebra T2. The spine of the scapula is approximately at T3. The inferior angle of the scapula and xiphoid process represent T7.

5. The answer is C.

Spina bifida occulta is a benign disorder. It presents with no decrease in function. There is no protrusion of the spinal cord or its associated structures, as in choices A and B.

6. The answer is A.

There are many benefits of exercise. Decreased HDL in answer A makes this an inappropriate list of the benefits of exercise. HDL is considered "good" cholesterol. Exercise decreases LDL and increases HDL in the bloodstream.

7. The answer is B.

Direct current is shown to have the greatest benefit in wound healing. Monophasic pulsed current has also been shown to have wound healing benefits.

8. The answer is D.

Choices A, B, and C would increase the functional length of the right lower extremity and possibly cause a circumduction during gait. Choice D would not change the functional leg length.

9. The answer is C.

A therapist can use ultrasound with all of the other choices. Performing an ultrasound over a cemented metal implant is also a contraindication. However, with any ultrasound technique, treatment should be stopped if the patient feels pain.

10. The answer is A.

The briefcase should be carried in the right hand. Carrying the briefcase in the left hand would increase the amount of force that the right gluteus medius would have to exert to maintain a stable pelvis during gait.

11. The answer is D.

Managers rated as 9,1 have high concern for productivity and low concern for employees. Managers classified as 5,5 have moderate concern for productivity and employees. Managers classified as 9,9 have a high concern for both. Managers rated as 1,9 have high concern for employees and little concern for productivity.

12. The answer is A.

A therapist's main responsibility with this patient is to maintain range of motion. Fluid retention is an important concern but for other medical staff. Choices C and D will be addressed later in the patient's course of therapy.

13. The answer is C.

The pitcher is moving into D2 extension with the throwing motion. He is strengthening the muscles involved in shoulder internal rotation, adduction, and forearm pronation.

14. The answer is B.

The iliofemoral ligament is the strongest ligament in the hip that prevents extension. It is the ligament most likely to be compromised in this scenario.

15. The answer is B.

Answers A and C are incorrect because rheumatoid arthritis is a contraindication for continuous or intermittent traction. Answer D is incorrect for the above reason as well as the fact that a 110-pound setting is too great for a 147-pound patient.

16. The answer is C.

Metatarsal pads successfully transfer weight onto the metatarsal shafts of this patient. A Thomas heel and a scaphoid pad are for patients with excessive pronation. A cushion heel absorbs shock at contact.

17. The answer is C.

Parkinson's disease and dementia are disorders involving the brain. Myasthenia gravis is a problem with acetylcholine receptors at the neuromuscular junction.

18. The answer is D.

Patellofemoral joint reaction forces increase as the angle of knee flexion and quadriceps muscle activity increase. Choice D involves the greatest knee flexion angle and quadriceps activity.

19. The answer is B.

A deficit in this region of the brain usually results in the inability to locate an extremity. This patient would have trouble putting on clothes.

20. The answer is A.

The danger in using a hot tub for a person with multiple sclerosis is that it may cause extreme fatigue. There is no need to avoid the other activities listed.

21. The answer is D.

A child with spastic diplegia most often presents with the lower extremities and trunk more involved than the upper extremities. Also one side is often more involved than the other side.

22. The answer is D.

In the ideal situation, the therapist should coordinate his or her plan of care with the chiropractor in case the problems are related.

23. The answer is B.

Grade I is a small oscillating movement at the beginning of range. Grade III is a large movement up to the end of available range. Grade IV is a small movement at the end of available range.

24. The answer is C.

Leaning the trunk over the involved hip decreases joint reaction force and strain on the hip abductors. These factors together decrease pain in the involved hip.

25. The answer is C.

A suberythemal dose of ultraviolet treatment is not enough to cause reddening of the skin. A minimal erythemal dose leads to slight itching and reddening. A third-degree erythemal dose is a more severe reaction with blister and edema formation.

26. The answer is C.

A physical therapist assistant (PTA) can do all of the listed options except change the frequency or duration as prescribed by a therapist or physician. Choice B allows the PTA to work within the protocol established by the physical therapist.

27. The answer is B.

Choice B describes fast-twitch muscle fibers. Choice A describes slow-twitch fibers. Choices C and D are incorrect answers.

28. The answer is C.

The lateral collateral ligament of the knee is best palpated with the patient in the sitting position. The patient then places the foot of the involved lower extremity on the knee of the uninvolved lower extremity. This maneuver places the involved knee in 90° of flexion and the hip in external rotation.

29. The answer is B.

The question describes a hemisection of the spinal cord, which is classified as a Brown-Sequard lesion. Anterior spinal cord injuries present with loss of motor function and insensitivity to pain and temperature bilaterally. Central cord injuries are characterized by loss of function in the upper extremities and normal function in the trunk and lower extremities.

30. The answer is D.

Choices A and B are correct exercise parameters for a healthy person. Choice B has the patient exercising at 65–90% of his age-adjusted maximal heart rate. Choice C is the patient's age-adjusted maximal heart rate.

31. The answer is B.

The patient is experiencing autonomic dysreflexia. The correct actions are to find the probable cause of the noxious stimulus and to lower the patient's blood pressure by inducing orthostatic hypotension. Patients with spinal cord injury above the level of T6 can experience this problem.

32. The answer is A.

Choice A is the correct postural drainage. Choice B is drained by resting on the right, ¼" turn to the back, and foot of the bed elevated 12–16 inches. Choices C and D are drained with patient in long sitting position or leaning forward over the pillow in sitting position.

33. The answer is A.

It is best to consult with the physician because of an extended amount of passive range of motion. A therapist should not deviate from a physician's order, but a telephone call to clarify the order is necessary when the therapist feels that another treatment plan is more appropriate.

34. The answer is C.

The therapist should notify the referring physician. The mistake should be documented and the patient informed. The referring physician can determine the need for a consultation with him or her or an obstetrician.

35. The answer is C.

Patients with recurrent ankle sprains benefit from proprioceptive exercises. Choices B and D are not indicated because of the lack of acute signs and symptoms. Choice A is a good plan, but not the most correct because there is no mention of proprioception.

36. The answer is B.

The patient can be successfully treated by using universal precautions. The patient should be treated in a relatively isolated area because of his weakened immune system. The diagnosis of AIDS with Kaposi's sarcoma is an indication that the patient's immune system is weak. Gloves should be used if the patient's sarcomas are open; otherwise, hand washing before and after patient contact is appropriate.

37. The answer is A.

A blood sugar value of 300 mg/dl is a contraindicated level for therapeutic exercise.

38. The answer is A.

I—No response. II—Generalized response. III—Localized responses. IV—Confused agitated. V—Confused inappropriate. VI—Confused appropriate. VII—Automatic appropriate. VIII—Purposeful and appropriate.

39. The answer is D.

An ulnar nerve-compromised hand presents as a "claw" hand after a prolonged amount of time because of atrophy of the interossei. The extensor digitorum takes over and pulls the MCPs in hyperextension.

40. The answer is B.

Bifid spinous processes (spinous processes that are split) are found only in the cervical spine.

41. The answer is A.

Local vasoconstriction is the first response. Nerve conduction velocity decreases after approximately 5 minutes of ice application.

42. The answer is B.

A lesion at choice A would cause bitemporal heteronymous hemianopsia. A lesion at choice C would cause left eye blindness, and a lesion at D would cause right eye blindness.

43. The answer is A.

A patient seriously injured in a hospital or a hospital-owned facility is a sentinel event. Other choices might be JCAHO violations, but only A is a sentinel event.

44. The answer is B.

The oburator nerve innervates the adductor brevis, adductor longus, adductor magnus, oburator externus, and gracilis muscles. Choice A has no motor function. Choice C innervates the sartorius, pectineus, iliacus, and quadriceps femoris. The ilioinguinal nerve innervates the obliquus internus abdominis and transversus abdominis.

45. The answer is B.

The patient should have made adequate progress in this period with this protocol. Because of the lack of progress, the patient needs further evaluation by the physician.

46. The answer is A.

Choice A is approximately 6–7 METs. Choice B is approximately 4.6 METs. Choice C is approximately 2 METs. Choice D is approximately 3–5 METs.

47. The answer is C.

Medicare Part A is used for inpatient treatment and Part B for outpatient treatment. Medicare part A or B can be used for home health treatment; part B being is when the patient does not have part A.

48. The answer is C.
Although sources vary widely, a child can sit unsupported usually between 4 and 8 months of age. Answers A and B are incorrect. Answer D would possibly cause the parent to worry prematurely.

49. The answer is A.
It is unethical to take gifts from anyone.

50. The answer is D.

Increased spasticity of the left gastrocnemius causes an increase in plantar flexion. Hypotonicity of the tibialis anterior causes a foot drop due to the inability to dorsiflex actively. A leg-length discrepancy should be evaluated in the initial assessment. This is a possibility in any patient, regardless of the diagnosis. The least likely cause of this deficit is a hypertonic left quadricep, which most likely would cause an increase in dorsiflexion on the involved side in an effort to decrease the functional leg length.

51. The answer is D.

The patient most likely has a rotator cuff tear. Choices A and B are incorrect because there is no need for heating modalities. Choice C is wrong because the patient has full passive range of motion; thus there is no need for stretching provided by the therapist at this point.

52. The answer is A.

A patient can obtain his or her medical records simply by signing a release form. Charts and records should never be given or faxed to an attorney unless the patient has signed a release.

53. The answer is D.

Choice D is the correct answer because A and B are the same type of study. The records of the factory are used to determine the frequency of disease. In a case-control study the people are selected based on whether or not they have a disease; then the frequency of the possible cause of the disease in the past is studied.

54. The answer is B.

A CORF is a classification of a type of outpatient facility.

55. The answer is A.

Choice A is the correct gait sequence for ascending stairs in the given scenario. A caregiver should stand below the patient because the patient is most likely to fall *down* the stairs. This same rule holds true for descending stairs.

56. The answer is B.

Hot packs are not indicated because there is no mention of abnormal muscle tone. The entire lumbar area is too much surface area for ultrasound. An argument could be made for lumbar traction, but it is paired with heating modalities in all of the answers.

57. The answer is A.

Ortolani's test is used to detect a congenitally dislocated hip in an infant. Choices B and C are common meniscus damage tests for the knee. Choice D is performed by placing the infant in supine position with the hip at 90° of flexion and slight abduction and the knee flexed to 90°. The examiner then moves the infant's hip anterior and posterior in an effort to detect abnormal joint mobility.

58. The answer is C.

Osgood-Schlatter disease is severe tendinitis of the patellar tendon. It is characterized by pronounced tibial tubercles. The increased size of the tubercles is attributed to the patella tendon pulling away from its insertion. Jumper's knees (or normal patella tendinitis) does not necessarily present with tubercle enlargement.

59. The answer is A.

Isometric exercises in the shortest range of the extensor muscle are used to begin strengthening. In contrast, weak flexor muscles should be strengthened in the middle-to-lengthened range, because they most often work near their end range.

60. The answer is A.

Choice A describes rheumatoid arthritis, a systemic condition. All of the other choices are signs and symptoms of osteoarthritis (OA). Sometimes OA can involve symmetrical joints, but it is not systemic.

61. The answer is B.

Choice B is the correct answer. Choice A is a posterior pelvic tilt.

62. The answer is C.

Dupuytren's contracture is a progressive thickening of the palmar aponeurosis of the hand. The progression is gradual, and the interphalangeal joints are pulled into flexion.

63. The answer is C.

In static standing the line of gravity is posterior to the hip joint. The body relies on the anterior pelvic ligaments and the hip joint capsule. The iliopsoas may be recruited at times, but anterior ligaments are used first to keep the trunk from extending in static stance.

64. The answer is C.

Answer B describes a swan-neck deformity.

65. The answer is C.

Mental status is the first item to assess. A therapist must first determine whether the patient is able to provide a reliable subjective history. It is also important to know whether the patient can follow a 1- or 2-step command before beginning a formal evaluation. The other choices should be assessed later in the evaluation.

66. The answer is A.

The therapist would use a PNF D1 diagonal to encourage the combined movements of hip flexion, adduction, and knee flexion. The diagonal also encourages the combined movements of hip adduction and extension. This is the combination of muscle activity most needed for gait.

67. The answer is C.

This scenario describes a central cord lesion. It is common in the geriatric population after cervical extension injuries (such as whiplash).

68. The answer is C.

Medicare requires that a patient living in a nursing home with Part A as the main source of reimbursement receive 5 days/week of skilled treatment. In this scenario, the physical therapist must see the patient 5 days/week because it is the only skilled service required by the patient.

69. The answer is A.

The lowest point in the gait cycle occurs when both lower extremities are in contact with the ground (double support).

70. The answer is C.

The patient's biological father would have the right to access the records whether or not he is on the list, but not the stepfather. Answer B is incorrect because unless he is on the original list, he cannot simply sign a form and receive the records. Answer D is incorrect because you cannot verify that you are speaking to the mother.

71. The answer is C.

Answer A is incorrect because the order is for occupational, not physical, therapy, and under that order the patient has to be treated by an occupational therapist. Answer B is incorrect because it is unlikely that a patient will agree to paying out of pocket or be able to afford the expense of occupational therapy services. Answer D is incorrect because the problem can be solved by telephone without making the patient schedule another doctor's appointment. Answer C is correct because it would take about 5 minutes to obtain a verbal order, and therapy can begin right away.

72. The answer is B.

Answer B is the most empathetic response. It also lets the patient know that the therapists will make an effort to prevent the problem from recurring.

73. The answer is C.

Answer A is incorrect because the patient should be able to learn how to be independent with activities of daily living. Answer B is incorrect because the patient can learn to drive an automobile independently with the assist of hand controls. Answer C is the correct answer because the patient may use momentum to negotiate a curb. Total balance of a wheelchair using a wheelie is an unrealistic goal.

74. The answer is A.

The screw home mechanism that is present in the last few degrees of terminal knee extension stresses the MCL. Sidelying hip adduction also places the MCL in a position of stretch.

75. The answer is D.

Answer A is incorrect because any way to solve this problem without denying needed therapy needs to be explored first. Answer B is incorrect because the therapist may be donating a considerable amount of time. This solution is not profitable for the therapist and is likely to cause an uncomfortable working atmosphere. Answer C is incorrect because the matter may be resolved without quitting. Answer D is correct because the immediate supervisor may be able to assist the therapist in coming to an agreement between the therapist and the company that employs them.

76. The answer is D.

This answer is correct because patients need a written home program with diagrams and instructions. One-on-one teaching is also necessary to ensure that the patient understands the program. Bringing in another family member is also definitely advisable to assist the patient with the program at home.

77. The answer is C.

The Joint Commission surveys hospitals once every 3 years.

78. The answer is B.

The area of contact between the humerus and the glenoid fossa is maximal in this position.

79. The answer is D.

This position places the least amount of stress on the lumbar spine in the sitting position.

80. The answer is D.

Performing isometric exercises places too much load on the left ventrical of the heart for many cardiac patients.

81. The answer is D.

These are signs and symptoms of a patient with bronchiectasis.

82. The answer is B.

A patient with a spinal cord injury at the C5 level would apply pressure to the abdomen to perform a cough. A patient with an injury at the T2 level and T10 level should be able to perform a cough independently, but this goal would be most challenging and obtainable for a patient with an injury at the level of C7.

83. The answer is D.

A belt that is angled at 90° with the sitting surface limits the patient's involuntary efforts to extend the trunk because of increased tone. This angle also allows the patient to actively tilt the pelvis anteriorly, which is a functional movement that does not need to be restricted.

84. The answer is D.

After the therapist assesses the patient for the first time, he or she needs to begin discharge planning. This is true for an assessment of any patient, not just in the inpatient rehabilitation setting.

85. The answer is B.

A fibers are the largest in diameter and conduct faster than C fibers.

86. The answer is D.

The subscapularis, teres minor, and infraspinatus muscles oppose the superior pull of the deltoid muscle. The supraspinatus does not oppose the pull of the deltoid but is important because (along with the other cuff muscles) it provides a compression force to the glenohumeral joint.

87. The answer is D.

Policies can be viewed as the rules, and procedures are the ways in which the rules are carried out.

88. The answer is A.

Only the edges of the adult meniscus are vascularized by the capillaries from the synovial membrane and joint capsule.

89. The answer is B.

The patient probably has a low left shoulder, prominent right scapula, and high left hip.

90. The answer is A.

Abdominal muscles attach to the lower border of the ribs and the superior surface of the pelvis. Strong abdominals prevent excessive anterior rotation of the pelvis during gait.

91. The answer is B.

D2 flexion patterns support upper trunk extension, which is important for patients with Parkinson's disease who tend to develop excessive kyphosis.

92. The answer is A.

Claudication is a lack of blood flow. This test is performed by having a patient walk on a treadmill and recording how long the patient can walk before the onset of claudication. Homan's sign is a test performed to see whether a patient may have a deep vein thrombosis. The percussion test is designed to assess the integrity of the greater saphoneous vein.

93. The answer is D.

The fastest settings are appropriate for isokinetic testing. A pitcher's throwing motion is quite fast. It is better to evaluate with the isokinetic speed as close as possible to the speed of the tested activity.

94. The answer is B.

A decreased tidal volume is caused by a restrictive lung dysfunction. An increased tidal volume is caused by an obstructive lung dysfunction.

95. The answer is C.

ST-segment displacement greater than 3 mm is a contraindication. Resting systolic pressure above 200 mmHg is a contraindication.

96. The answer is B.

A rating of 9 corresponds with "very light." A rating of 7 is "very, very light." A rating of 13 is "somewhat hard." A rating of 15 is "hard." A rating of 17 is "very hard." A rating of 19 is "very, very hard."

97. The answer is D.

Choices A and C provide the most medial/lateral ankle support. A posterior leaf-spring ankle-foot orthosis only provides assistance with dorsiflexion.

98. The answer is D.

Dexamethasone is a common anti-inflammatory drug driven with the negative electrode. Lidocaine is a commonly used analgesic driven with the positive electrode.

99. The answer is A.

The intervertebral disc has the greatest amount of fluid at the time of birth. The fluid content decreases as a person ages.

100. The answer is A.

In the case of a reciprocal click, the initial click is created by the condyle slipping back into the correct position under the disk with opening of the mouth. In this disorder, the condyle is resting posterior to the disk before jaw opening. With closing the click is caused by the condyle slipping away from the disk.

101. The answer is D.

The supraspinatus tendon is best palpated by placing the patient's involved upper extremity behind the back in full internal rotation.

102. The answer is A.

The plantar calcaneonavicular ligament originates on the sustentaculum tali of the calcaneus and inserts on the navicular. This ligament, along with the long plantar ligament, plantar aponeurosis, and the short plantar ligament, gives support to the longitudinal arch of the foot. Choice A is the most important ligament.

103. The answer is B.

The fifth lumbar nerve root is impinged because it arises from the spinal column superior to the L4–L5 lumbar disc.

104. The answer is B.

This gait deviation is caused by the patient leaning back to decrease the flexion moment created at the hip at initial contact. The gluteus maximus is most responsible for counteracting this flexion moment.

105. The answer is C.

This set of signs and symptoms most likely points to multiple sclerosis. The other conditions listed are progressive, but the best answer is multiple sclerosis.

106. The answer is D.

Compression stockings (e.g., Jobst, TED hose) are used in patients with poor venous return. A patient with chronic arterial disease already has difficulty with getting blood to the lower extremities; there is no need to further inhibit the flow.

107. The answer is D.

The correct treatment involves debridement of the eschar over the wound. Elase is an enzymatic wound debridement ointment. Lidocaine is an anesthetic. Dexamethasone is a steroid used mainly with iontophoresis. Silvadene is an antimicrobial used to prevent infection.

108. The answer is D.

Exercising at the peak time of insulin effect causes hypoglycemia. Insulin causes the liver to decrease sugar production. The body needs increased levels of blood glucose during exercise.

109. The answer is C.

A curve greater than 120° is often associated with restrictive lung dysfunction. The other factors listed are not life-threatening.

110. The answer is A.

These signs are consistent with restrictive lung dysfunction.

111. The answer is B.

The responses of the patient represent the lowest possible score on the Glasgow Coma Scale. One point is given for each of the listed responses (or lack thereof).

112. The answer is D.

These signs and symptoms are consistent with an injury to the anterior cerebral artery.

113. The answer is C.

This answer is correct because the most common deformity after a severe burn such as this is hip flexion, hip adduction, knee flexion, and ankle plantar flexion.

114. The answer is B.

With a disagreement about treatment, the therapist should speak with the physician directly.

115. The answer is D.

The therapist should meet with the nephew on his or her own time and review the exercises.

116. The answer is B.

The supervisor can best handle this situation by discussing the exercise program away from the patient. Correcting the new graduate in front of the patient probably would decrease the confidence of the patient in the treatment and the therapist.

117. The answer is A.

An electric wheelchair definitely uses less energy but does not require the physical effort needed by this patient to maintain functional mobility. Ambulation with a knee-ankle-foot orthosis is probably possible but requires much more energy than locomotion with a manual wheelchair. Ankle-foot orthoses alone do not provide enough support for the patient to attempt ambulation.

118. The answer is A.

This theory supports the use of a TENS unit for sensory level pain control. The activation of the larger fibers decreases the amount of sensory information traveling to the brain.

119. The answer is A.

Choice A probably would activate increased tone because of the resistance to plantar flexion offered by the spring.

120. The answer is D.

The metacarpophalangeal joint is enclosed in a joint capsule and therefore is considered a diarthrodial joint.

121. The answer is A.

A defect in the lamina of a vertebrae usually occurs first. This defect is called spondylolysis. The vertebrae may then slip because of shear forces; this slippage is called spondylolisthesis.

122. The answer is C.

The therapist must stretch the inferior portion of the capsule in an effort to gain abduction of the involved shoulder. This principle is supported by the convex-concave rule.

123. The answer is C.

The superior pole is in most contact at approximately 90° of knee flexion.

124. The answer is A.

Atherthrombotic strokes are caused by blood clots in the brain. Atherosclerosis leads to blood clots.

125. The answer is B.

Choice B best describes the position that causes injury only to the ACL. In most cases an audible pop indicates a tear of the ACL. Varus or valgus blows to the knee injure the collateral ligaments and possibly the ACL.

126. The answer is B.

Rheumatoid arthritis is a systemic condition commonly involving joints bilaterally. Crepitus can be associated with osteoarthritis or rheumatoid arthritis, but rheumatoid arthritis is the most likely in this case.

127. The answer is C.

The "painful arc" is most indicative of shoulder impingement. The soft tissues of the shoulder are pinched under the acromion process at approximately 60–120° of abduction. Pain throughout abduction active range of motion suggests acromioclavicular joint dysfunction.

128. The answer is D.

These signs and symptoms are most likely associated with damage to the cerebellum. Injuries to the basal ganglia can present with the following symptoms: rigidity, resting tremor, choreiform movements (jerky movements), and difficulty with initiating movement. Frontal lobe lesions lead to a change in mood or overall personality. The dorsal columns are involved in proprioception and awareness of movement.

129. The answer is D.

The lateral triangle (composed of the radial head, olecranon process, and lateral epicondyle) is the most likely of the choices to exhibit joint edema. Joint edema is common after a surgical procedure.

130. The answer is B.

To prevent pressure (decubitis) ulcers effectively, patients should be turned every 2 hours.

131. The answer is A.

A platelet count of 45,000 is low, but a count of approximately 20,000 is considered a contraindication for percussion treatment. Normal values are above 260,000.

132. The answer is D.

Riding a stationary bike at 5.5 mph is approximately 3.5 METs. Descending a flight of stars is approximately 4–5 METs. Ironing is approximately 3.5 METs. Ambulating 5–6 mph is approximately 8.6 METs.

133. The answer is B.

The correct procedure is answer B. Subtracting 1 inch allows correct pressure distribution over the patient's buttocks and thighs.

134. The answer is B.

During pregnancy a woman normally experiences an increase in resting heart rate and a decrease in heart rate during exercise. This change is compared with the heart rate of the particular woman before pregnancy. The other answers are true about pregnancy.

135. The answer is D.

One of the main reasons that pelvic floor exercises are beneficial for a pregnant woman is the extra weight of the viscera.

136. The answer is C.

Posting the inservice date on the bulletin board and sending a memo to the department heads is the most effective way to invite everyone interested. Scheduling during lunch often makes it easier for people to attend.

137. The answer is C.

A burst fracture causes damage to the spinal cord because bony fragments are pushed posteriorly into the spinal canal. This type of fracture is often accompanied with anterior cord syndrome.

138. The answer is D.

The Thomas test is a screen to determine whether the hip flexors are too tight.

139. The answer is B.

A therapist should never comment on such a serious prognosis before the physician has assessed the lab results and consulted with the patient first.

140. The answer is D.

To assist a patient in developing a tenodesis grip, the therapist should allow the patient's finger flexors to tighten. This grip functions with active extension of the wrist, which allows flexion of the fingers because of shortened flexor tendons.

141. The answer is A.

The symptoms involving the left lower extremity are an indication that a disc is herniated or protruding onto a nerve root on the left side. A positive straight leg-raise test is also often an indication of a disc herniation or protrusion.

142. The answer is C.

This answer is the most appropriate. The therapist cannot guarantee everything will be okay (answer A) or that the physician is the best (answer B). Answer D is too insensitive.

143. The answer is B.

A socket that is too large may cause the prosthetic limb to "drop" during ambulation.

144. The answer is C.

The foot drop is caused by a lack of active dorsiflexion. The tibilias anterior is responsible for this motion and is innervated by the deep peroneal nerve.

145. The answer is C.

Adson's maneuver tests for thoracic outlet syndrome. Lhermitte's sign tests for dural irritation in the cervical spine.

146. The answer is A.

The anterior surface of the face and the upper extremity are each considered 4.5% of the body, according to the rule of nines. The anterior trunk is 18%. Each anterior surface of the lower extremities is 9%. The posterior side is the same, respectively. The total groin area is 1%.

147. The answer is C.

The axis point is the knee joint. The effort arm is distal to the knee joint at the insertion of the patella tendon. The resistance is at the ankle. A class-two lever has the resistance arm in the middle, making a longer effort arm than resistance arm. The class-one lever has an axis in the middle.

148. The answer is D.

A superficial partial-thickness burn and a deep partial-thickness burn are not deep enough to involve the subcutaneous tissue. An electrical burn is complete destruction of the subcutaneous tissue. A full-thickness burn produces moderate subcutaneous tissue damage and little pain.

149. The answer is B.

According to the American Heart Association, a person is determined unresponsive before emergency medical service is activated.

150. The answer is D.

A shuffling gait and difficulty with initiating gait are typical signs of Parkinson's disease.

151. The answer is C.

The pelvis is dropping on the right side because the left gluteus medius is weak. The patient also may lean toward the left hip joint to move the center of gravity, making it easier to hold up the right side of the pelvis.

152. The answer is C.

This is called Ober's test, which screens for a tight iliotibial band.

153. The answer is D.

The involved upper extremity is in this position because of damage to the C5 and C6 spinal roots.

154. The answer is C.

Rhythmic stabilization involves a series of isometric contractions of the agonist, then the antagonist.

155. The answer is D.

Choice D describes an expiratory reserve volume. Choice A is residual volume, choice B is tidal volume, and choice C is vital capacity.

156. The answer is C.

Choice C describes the symmetric tonic neck reflex. With passive cervical extension an infant displays upper extremity extension and lower extremity flexion.

157. The answer is A.

Infants accomplish this task between approximately 5 and 10 months of age. The response in choice A would prevent the parent from excessive unnecessary worry. Sources vary widely about the exact month when developmental milestones are reached, but A is the correct answer in this scenario.

158. The answer is D.

If the foot is outset too much, it is likely to cause the prosthetic knee to bow inward during standing.

159. The answer is C.

The right lower extremity is still strong, and there is no facial droop or diminished sensation. Although these signs are not always present after a stroke, the other signs and symptoms, such as a history of a recent fall and the past total hip replacement, should lead the therapist to choice C. The patient cannot lift the right lower extremity in the standing position because it increases weight-bearing on the fractured left lower extremity. The left leg also shows a definite strength loss as graded with manual muscle testing.

160. The answer is A.

Choice A describes an isotonic exercise. Choice B is an isometric exercise. Choice C is an isokinetic exercise.

161. The answer is D.

Dry skin is a sign of a diabetic coma.

162. The answer is D.

The white cell count in a patient with this diagnosis would decrease. Lupus affects mostly young women.

163. The answer is D.

Hypertension is a risk factor in atherosclerosis.

164. The answer is D.

A stratified random sample is taken by dividing the test population into two groups or strata (in this case, male and female) and taking a random sample from each group.

165. The answer is C.

The physical therapist should tell the assistant to wait until they can both work together with the patient. The family is not qualified to help the assistant during the first attempt at ambulation in this situation.

166. The answer is B.

This form of spina bifida is associated with direct involvement with the cauda equina. The muscles that are innervated by the cauda equina usually present with flaccid paralysis.

167. The answer is A.

Torticollis involving the right sternocleidomastoid would cause right lateral cervical flexion and left cervical rotation.

168. The answer is D.

A positive Tinel's sign screens for carpal tunnel syndrome when the tapping force is performed over the carpal tunnel itself. In Phalen's test, the therapist places the patient's wrists in maximal flexion and holds for 1 minute. The test is positive if there is parasthesia in the median nerve distribution. The Finkelstein test screens for de Quervain's disease by allowing the patient to make a fist with the thumb wrapped in the fingers. The test is positive if there is pain over the adbuctor pollicis longus and extensor pollicis brevis tendons.

169. The answer is D.

Tissue with a high collagen content absorbs more ultrasound. Bone absorbs the most ultrasound.

170. The answer is C.

Answers A, B, and D increase heart rate. Quinidine is an antiarrhythmic drug.

171. The answer is D.

A myocardial infarction that involves the left ventricle is likely to cause cardiogenic shock. Cardiogenic shock is a rapid decline in cardiac output. Vascular shock is widespread vasodilation. Toxic and anaphylactic shock occur when the body is exposed to a toxin or allergin, respectively.

172. The answer is C.

The capitate is the axis.

173. The answer is A.

The ADA allowed structural modifications of federal buildings and protection from discrimination based on disability.

174. The answer is B.

A patient with damage to Broca's area is a right hemiplegic. Damage to this area causes difficulty with speaking and sometimes difficulty with writing. Usually damage to this area does not impair the ability to understand written or spoken language.

175. The answer is D.

This is a description of a CT scan. A PET scan is performed by injecting a radioactive compound into the person being tested and then forming a picture of the brain with a computer that picks up the compound that reaches the brain tissue. An MRI picks up radiofrequency waves that are emitted by atomic particles displaced by radio waves in a magnetic field. An angiogram uses a high contrast dye that reveals the vessels of the brain by x-ray.

176. The answer is B.

The person should lie down to prevent head injury. Tight clothes are loosened to make sure that nothing is too constricting. Close furniture is moved away for the patient's safety. Nothing should be placed in the patient's mouth because of the danger of obstructing the airway.

177. The answer is B.

Answer A is a description of a McGregor Theory Y Manager. Answer C is an example of William Ouchi's Theory Z. Answer D is part of the thought behind Herzberg's Two-Factor Theory.

178. The answer is C.

Tetralogy of Fallot consists of these four abnormalities.

179. The answer is B.

Genu valgum is a term used to describe a deformity of the knee causing an inward bowing of the legs. Genu varus is an outward bowing of the legs. Coxa valgum is a deformity at the hip in which the angle between the axis of the neck of the femur and the shaft of the femur is greater than 135°. In coxa varus this angle is less than 135°. Pes cavus is an increase in the arch of the foot. Pes planus is flat foot.

180. The answer is C.

This is the loose-packed position of the hip.

181. The answer is A.

The second cuneiform of the foot articulates with the first cuneiform, second metatarsal, third cuneiform, and navicular.

182. The answer is D.

A person in a diabetic coma has low blood pressure.

183. The answer is A.

Metatarsal pads, metatarsal bars, and rocker bars transfer weight onto the metatarsal shaft. A scaphoid pad is for patients with excessive pronation.

184. The answer is B.

Exercise testing should be terminated at 2 mm of ST depression.

185. The answer is D.

This type of orthotic uses tenodesis to achieve opening and closing of the hand. To close the hand, the patient actively extends the wrist. To open the hand, the patient passively flexes the wrist.

186. The answer is D.

A person with spastic quadriplegia presents with talipes equinovarus. This term is synonymous with clubfoot.

187. The answer is A.

This is a description of a first-degree atrioventricular block. The heart rate is usually between 60 and 100 beats/minute.

188. The answer is D.

To lock the elbow with this type of prosthesis, the patient must extend the humerus and depress the scapula.

189. The answer is A.

Any phrase stated by the patient that is relevant information goes into the subjective portion of the note.

190. The answer is C.

Neurapraxia is not associated with axon degeneration; it is associated instead with demyelination and complete recovery. With axonotmesis there is wallerian degeneration below the site of the lesion. In neurotmesis the damage is so severe that full function may not be regained.

191. The answer is C.

A score of one is given for each of the following: some resistance of the extremities to movement, a heart rate less than 100 beats/minute, and slow respirations. A score of zero is given for bluish color in the body and extremities and no response to reflex irritability.

192. The answer is B.

In performing contract-relax-contract antagonist in this particular situation, the internal rotators are actively contracted first; the external rotators are contracted next in an effort to increase external range of motion. The agonists are the internal rotators (tight muscle group in this situation), and the antagonists are the external rotators. The infraspinatus, teres minor, and supraspinatus assist the external rotators. The subscapularis is an internal rotator. Other larger muscles also participate in rotation, but this question refers to the rotator cuff muscles.

193. The answer is C.

Patients with congestive heart failure often develop an enlarged heart because of the burden of an increased preload and afterload.

194. The answer is A.

Leukocytes respond to an injury by emigrating into the blood stream. The next step of the leukocytes is margination, which is movement toward the inner surface of the vessels.

195. The answer is D.

The five stages of grieving are (in order from first to last) denial, anger, bargaining, depression, and acceptance.

196. The answer is C.

The common peroneal nerve travels over the lateral knee. It is the *least* likely to be injured. The other structures are either within the knee or directly posterior.

197. The answer is B.

Asking prospective employees how many children they have is inappropriate.

198. The answer is C.

Because the patient does not have 50% of normal range of motion in the gravity eliminated position, 2–/5 is the appropriate grade. Some therapists argue that this is an example of a 1+/5 grade. Sources used in preparation of this exam indicate that there is no grade of 1+/5 with manual muscle testing.

199. The answer is D.

The ACL-deficient patient has a significant rotatory instability. Bracing may prevent some of this instability. Sports that are especially difficult on the knees (e.g., skiing, competitive tennis) are contraindicated.

200. The answer is C.

Correct electrode placement is over the motor points of the involved muscle. On–off cycle time is usually between 1:3 and 1:5. Fused tetany of a muscle usually occurs between 50–80 hertz or pps (sources vary).

201. The answer is D.

Choice D is the correct answer because in the supine position the abdominal contents are located more superiorly than in the other positions. This places the diaphragm in a more elevated resting position, which allows greater excursion of the diaphragm. Semi-Fowler's position resembles a reclining position, with the knees bent and the upper trunk slightly elevated. Semi-Folwer's position, without an abdominal binder, allows gravity to pull the abdominal contents downward, which does not put the diaphragm in an optimal resting position. Semi-Fowler's position is, however, the position of choice for patients with uncompromised innervation of the diaphragm who have chronic respiratory difficulty. The standing and sitting positions present the same problem, but to a greater extent, as semi-Fowler's position.

202. The answer is D.

The pressure applied by the therapist should be applied as the patient coughs to assist in a forceful exhalation. Placing the heel of one hand approximately one inch above the umbilicus applies pressure immediately inferior to the diaphragm.

203. The answer is B.

Physical therapists can assist a patient with dysarthria and dysphagia by (1) providing posture control exercises for the head and trunk, which assist the effectiveness of the respiration muscles in providing air volume for vocalization; (2) providing exercises for the facial musculature, including the lips and tongue, to assist in vocalization; (3) providing effective verbal interaction with the patient; and (4) minimizing any unnecessary stimuli or distractions during physical therapy sessions. The speech therapist is most qualified to work with the patient on swallowing techniques for liquids and solids.

204. The answer is B.

Use of a sliding board is the most functional transfer for this patient. The pneumatic lift requires assistance from another person, on which this patient can rely because he lives alone and has poor outside family support. A fully reclined geriatric chair is often used to transfer obese patients with a slide sheet transfer, which requires two or more people. A trapeze bar may be useful, but transferring wheelchair to bed with a sliding board teaches the patient the skill needed to transfer from the wheelchair to many other surfaces (that may not have a trapeze bar to assist).

205. The answer is C.

Raynaud's phenomenon is a vasospastic disorder of the vessels of the distal parts of the extremities. Patients with Raynaud's phenomenon do not respond well to cold treatment. Choice B is incorrect because it is believed that moist heat may encourage more rapid growth of cancer. Choice D is incorrect because prolonged use of steroids may cause capillaries to lose their integrity, which compromises the body's ability to dissipate heat. Choice A is incorrect because moist heat may encourage hemorrhaging, in patients with hemophilia by causing vasodilation.

206. The answer is B.

Although the change may be minimal, increasing the maximal pressure to 60 mmHg is the most likely choice to have a positive affect on edema reduction. The pressure, however, should not exceed the diastolic pressure of the patient. Answer A is not the right choice because placing the extremity in a dependent position causes the pump to work against gravity. Answer C is an incorrect choice because decreasing the on time means that the extremity receives compression for a shorter period. Answer D is an incorrect choice because greater pressure distally is more likely to move fluid than equal pressure throughout the sleeve.

207. The answer is D.

The fingers can be bound in paraffin wax as well as in fluidotherapy. When using this technique, the hand remains stationary throughout the heating process, which is necessary for paraffin to be most effective (when using the standard method of dipping the hand and wrapping with plastic wrap and a towel).

208. The answer is B.

Viscosity is the friction of fluids. Buoyancy is the property that pushes up on the part immersed with a pressure that is equal to the weight of the amount of water displaced by that part. Relative density states that if the specific gravity of an object is less than one it will float and if it is greater than one it will sink. Hydrostatic pressure is the property of water that places pressure equally on the immersed part.

209. The answer is B.

Answer A is true because near-infrared can penetrate up to 10 mm compared with 2 mm with far-infrared. Answer B is a false statement because infrared lamps can heat only one side of an extremity at a time. Answers C and D are true statements because the intensity of the infrared can be changed by altering the angle of the beam with the treated part or the distance between the body part and the lamp.

210. The answer is C.

Answer C provides correct instructions. The patient is often instructed to begin this technique in the supine position and progress to the sitting position. This technique should be practiced for approximately 5 minutes several times per day.

211. The answer is B.

Although a stroke may have occurred, the physical therapist can first evaluate and treat the patient. After the evaluation has been performed, the therapist will be more informed about the patient's condition and can then contact the physician if necessary.

212. The answer is A.

Back blows should be followed by chest thrusts with complete airway obstruction when CPR is performed on an infant. The therapist then should check for a foreign body in the airway. A blind finger sweep of the throat should not be performed on an infant.

213. The answer is D.

The Romberg test is a type of equilibrium test. Equilibrium tests are usually conducted with the patient in a standing position, whereas nonequilibrium tests are performed with the patient in the supine position.

214. The answer is A.

The signs and symptoms are consistent with a patient in the acute stage of RSD. Dystrophic signs and symptoms are decreased temperature, cessation of hair and nail growth, pale skin, and muscle atrophy. Atrophic signs and symptoms are decreased hypersensitivity, normal temperature, marked muscle atrophy, and smooth skin.

215. The answer is C.

Trigger points are often treated with soft tissue massage. Other techniques include strain/counterstrain, myofascial release, and muscle energy techniques.

216. The answer is A.

Patients with ideomotor apraxia often can identify objects but cannot use them correctly on command. Such patients often can perform the activity spontaneously. Patients with ideational apraxia often cannot identify objects or use them. Both situations call for short one-step commands.

217. The answer is A.

As perception improves, objects should be moved into the area of the deficit (the right side in this case), but initially they should be placed in plain view of the patient (the left side in this case).

218. The answer is C.

Fully elevating the leg rests of the patient's chair increases hip flexion. The already tight hamstrings (secondary to contracture) would tilt the pelvis posterior. This maneuver would increase weight on the ischial tuberosity, risking a decubitus ulcer. Choice D is correct advice because sliding board transfers can lead to abrasions. Choices A and B are also correct measures to decrease the chance of developing ulcers.

219. The answer is D.

The geriatric population usually has a decreased body temperature due to poor diet, decreased cardiovascular status, and decreased metabolic rates.

220. The answer is B.

The sedentary patient's cardiovascular response increases faster than the trained patient's if the workloads are equal.

221. The answer is D.

Answer A is contraindicated because the electromagnetic field produced by use of short-wave diathermy or microwave diathermy may alter the settings of a pacemaker. Answer B is contraindicated because the metal heats quickly and may cause the surrounding tissue to heat excessively, potentially causing a burn. Answer C is contraindicated because heating causes vasodilation, making a hemorrhage more likely. Answer D is the correct choice because pulsed short-wave diathermy can be used on acute or chronic conditions. With most pulsed short-wave treatments there is no measurable temperature increase in the tissues.

222. The answer is C.

The EMG does not record torque. It assists by showing a linear relationship between the EMG and the force produced by the muscle during an isometric contraction.

223. The answer is C.

Placing a plug-in unit close to water pipes is a potential hazard because it offers another possible ground pathway to the patient. Never use an extension cord or an adaptor with a plug-in unit. If the adaptor or cord does not have a ground prong, it may cause shock to the patient through a leaking current. If the machine intensity is adjusted during the off portion of the cycle, the stimulation may be too high for the patient when the on cycle returns.

224. The answer is B.

This is an example of a bipolar configuration. Another form of bipolar configuration is to have two electrodes of equal size, each from a different lead wire. In a monopolar configuration, one smaller electrode is placed over the intended site and a larger electrode is placed some distance away. The stimulation is perceived by the patient, in this case, only under the smaller electrode. In a quadripolar configuration, two electrodes coming from two different lead wires are placed over the intended area.

225. The answer is B.

Answer B is correct because the patient has to achieve passive knee extension before she can gain full active knee extension. Full active knee extension and full flexion are important and should be a major focus of the patient's session, but the question asks for the most serious deficit. Ambulating with a lesser assistive device should be the focus at a later time because the patient's gait is still severely antalgic and obvious instability is still present. Usually a patient is advanced to a lesser assistive device when he or she can ambulate without large gait deviations with the current assistive device.

226. The answer is C.

Answer C is incorrect. Heat decreases spasm by causing the vessels to dilate, which brings more blood (containing oxygen) to the area. Cold decreases spasm by decreasing sensitivity of the muscle spindles.

227. The answer is C.

Because of the unreliable history obtained in the evaluation, the therapist at least should make a quick assessment of range of motion and strength before the patient attempts to stand. Sit-to-stand transfer should then be assessed in front of the lift chair before the patient attempts to ambulate.

228. The answer is D.

This sequence assists in propelling the center of gravity forward to maintain balance after a backward sway.

229. The answer is B.

The Barthel Index assesses 10 self-care and mobility areas (including locomotion). The score is based on the amount of time and assistance required to perform a task. The Kenny Self-Care Evaluation measures 17 basic activities of daily living and grades from 0 to 4 (totally dependent to independent). The Katz Index measures 6 basic activities of daily living but does not measure wheelchair mobility or ambulation skills. The Functional Status Index measures the patient's opinion about how much pain is involved with an activity, how much assistance he or she requires to perform a task, and his or her dependence level.

230. The answer is D.

More than 10% of polyphasic potentials in the total output of muscle is considered abnormal.

231. The answer is C.

In performing these tests on patients who have a motor neuron disease, sensory potentials are generally unchanged.

232. The answer is C.

Because the hip flexors are strong, there is no need for the hip component of an orthotic.

233. The answer is A.

Before a job-site analysis can begin, the therapist should be familiar with the injuries or problems occurred at the job-site and the employee's job description.

234. The answer is D.

The hip strategy is used to compensate for large movements in the center of mass, and the ankle strategy is used to compensate for small movements.

235. The answer is D.

The first sound heard corresponds with closing of the mitral and tricuspid valves. The second sound corresponds to closing of the aortic and pulmonic valves. Therefore, the first sound is indicative of the onset of ventricular systole, and the second sound is indicative of the onset of ventricular diastole.

236. The answer is C.

The difference in measurements suggests a pelvic imbalance, which often is seen in patents who have scoliosis. Answers A and B would have exhibited differences in real leg length (anterior superior iliac spine to the medial malleolus).

237. The answer is C.

The Joint Commission on Accreditation of Healthcare Organizations requires at least one-yearly inspection of electrical equipment.

238. The answer is A.

A ground fault interruption circuit protects the patient from a potentially life-threatening situation. The other choices are valid concerns, but A is the most important.

239. The answer is B.

Pressure on the left temporal bone just anterior to the ear helps to occlude blood flow from the temporal artery.

240. The answer is A.

A patient of this age usually can begin with crutches instead of a standard walker. If the patient has no cognitive deficits and was independent in ambulation without an assistive device before surgery, she most likely will have the balance and coordination necessary to ambulate with crutches. A three-point gait pattern is necessary because of the current partial weight-bearing status. A swing-to pattern also can be used, but a three-point pattern assists more quickly in returning a more normal gait pattern.

241. The answer is C.

The therapist should never instruct a patient to change the dosage of the medication. In addition, calling the physician and expressing concerns about the possible effects of the medication observed at therapy would be much more appropriate than calling to suggest another medication.

242. The answer is A.

The method used in answer A is the safest. The method used in answer C is too unstable.

243. The answer is A.

Barognosis is the ability to differentiate between different weights. Stereognosis is the ability to differentiate between different sizes and shapes. Graphesthesia is the ability to identify letters, numbers, or designs traced on the skin. Texture recognition is the ability to differentiate between textures such as cotton, wool, and silk.

244. The answer is A.

The patient is using palmar prehension in this scenario. Palmar prehension is holding an object between the thumb pad and the middle and index finger. Fingertip prehension is used when a person picks up an object between the thumb pad and either the index or middle finger (not both at the same time, as with palmar prehension). In lateral prehension, the thumb pad is in contact with the lateral side of the index finger proximal to the distal interphalangeal joint. In hook grasp, the fingers are flexed as if carrying a bucket by the handle. The thumb does not provide much active movement when the hook grasp is used.

245. The answer is A.

Patients with decerebrate rigidity are positioned with all extremities extended, and the wrist and fingers flexed. Patients with decorticate posturing are positioned with the upper extremities flexed, the lower extremities hyperextended, and the fingers tightly flexed.

246. The answer is B.

The mean is the average of the set of numbers. The mode is the number that appears most often in the set of data. The median is the middlemost value.

247. The answer is D.

Men with high complete lesions are likely to be able to have reflexogenic erections, and men with lower complete lesion are likely to have the capability to have a reflexogenic or psychogenic erection. Men with incomplete lesions are likely to retain erectile capability much more than men with complete lesions. In addition, a man with a complete lesion is less likely to have the ability to ejaculate than a man with an incomplete lesion.

248. The answer is C.

Patients with chronic obstructive airway disease are often given this set of instructions, which is known as the method of pursed lips breathing. This method helps a patient regain control of his or her breathing rate and increase tidal volume and amount of oxygen absorbed.

249. The answer is C.

This is a description of the petrissage technique. Effleurage is stroking of the skin. Friction massages are used to mobilize scar tissue. Tapotement is tapping of the skin.

250. The answer is D.

Dermatome charts in distribution vary from source to source, but one common aspect of C7 innervation is the middle finger. The triceps muscles are also innervated by C7.

251. The answer is B.

Iontophoresis uses direct current to drive medication through the skin by repelling ions. For example, if a medication is positively charged, it can be driven by the anode (the positive electrode); if a medication is negatively charged, it can be driven by the cathode (the negative electrode).

252. The answer is A.

AIDS is transmitted by blood or bodily fluids. Masks are usually used with airborne precautions. Handwashing should be done between all wound care patients. Gloves are also indicated with all open wounds. Gowns may not be a necessity but should be used if there is a chance of soiling the clothing with infected fluids.

253. The answer is A.

A step stool decreases the overall shoulder elevation required. Answer B increases shoulder elevation, and answer C maintains internal rotation with increased elevation. External rotation with elevation decreases the impingement to the rotator cuff muscles.

254. The answer is B.

Because the goals were not completed in a short amount of time, a new long-term goal should be set. Because of the significant progress made in outpatient therapy, there is no need to return to the rehabilitation unit.

255. The answer is D.

All of the choices are important, but the dietary assessment contains the least amount of critical information at this stage of the physical therapy evaluation.

256. The answer is D.

Dialysis leads to a change in blood chemistry and volume, often causing extreme fatigue.

257. The answer is D.

During a functional capacity evaluation the physical therapist should not correct postural abnormalities. The therapist should only observe and record.

258. The answer is B.

Passive extension is the most important motion to gain after an anterior cruciate ligament reconstruction, regardless of the graft type. Active extension can be achieved once passive extension is full (or equal bilaterally).

259. The answer is A.

Because the patient lives alone, independent transfer is the most important goal listed. Functional ambulation is an important goal, but choice B is an unrealistic goal for the patient to accomplish in a 2- or 3-day period.

260. The answer is D.

When a patient with Parkinson's disease has been using levodopa for an extended period, he or she may develop resistance to the medication. Sometimes a break from the drug for 7–10 days may enhance its effectiveness.

261. The answer is A.

Normal hematocrit values for women are 36–48%; for men, 40–52%.

262. The answer is C.

Supine positioning without a pillow under the knees places too much stress on the lumbar spine. Sidelying position with a pillow between the knees places less stress on the lumbar area than prone positioning.

263. The answer is C.

This scenario describes a greenstick fracture, which is common in young people. In a comminuted fracture, the bone is broken into pieces. An example of an avulsion fracture is when the tibial tuberosity is pulled off the tibia. A bone that has a segmental fracture is fractured in two places.

264. The answer is D.

All of the listed muscles participate in mandibular elevation with the exception of the lateral pterygoid muscle. The lateral pterygoid muscle and the suprahyoid muscles participate in mandibular depression.

265. The answer is D.

This is an example of an associated reaction, which presents from birth to 3 months and is integrated at 9 years of age. The Landau reaction (onset at 4 months, integrated at 24 months) is assessed by supporting the patient in prone position and passively or actively extending the neck. A positive response is extension of the spine and lower extremities. The startle reflex is positive if an infant is startled by a loud or sudden noise. This response should be present at birth and persists throughout life. The Moro reflex is tested by lowering an infant suddenly from a sitting position. A positive response is crying with sudden extension and abduction of the upper extremities, followed by adduction of the upper extremities across the chest (an infant should have this response up to 6 months of age). Sources vary significantly in regard to the age at which these responses should be present and when they are integrated.

266. The answer is D.

The Moro reflex and the Landau reaction are discussed in the answer to question 265. Labyrinthine head-righting is tested by holding a child upright and tilting the body slightly forward, back, and side to side. The infant should be able to hold the head vertical despite the body movement. The symmetric tonic neck response (onset at 4–6 months, integrated at 8–12 months) is exhibited when the infant displays upper extremity extension and lower extremity flexion with passive cervical extension. Sources vary significantly in regard to the age at which these responses should be present and when they are integrated.

267. The answer is B.

A person with C4 quadriplegia can be reasonably expected to use a power wheelchair for locomotion with mouth, chin, breath, or sip-and-puff controls. A person with C5 quadriplegia may be reasonably expected to be able to transfer independently from wheelchair to bed with a sliding board. A person with C4 quadriplegia may be able to feed independently but will need some type of assistive device. A person with C5 quadriplegia may be able to don a shirt with assistance. Sources vary significantly on this subject.

268. The answer is B.

A person with C7 quadriplegia should be able to use a wheelchair without power controls. The goals set in answers A and D do not represent the maximal functional potential for this patient. The goal in answer C is set too high for this patient.

269. The answer is B.

This goal should be most challenging and obtainable for a patient with C7 quadriplegia. A person with C4 or C5 quadriplegia probably needs assistance from another person to dress and bathe. A person with C7 quadriplegia would find this goal more challenging than a person with T1 paraplegia.

270. The answer is C.

A person is usually diagnosed with type I at 25 years of age or younger. A person is usually 40 years of age or older when diagnosed with type II. Ketoacidosis is a symptom of type I. Metabolism of free fatty acids in the liver causes this condition which is an excess of ketones. A type II diabetic may be able to control his or her condition with diet only (depending on the severity of the condition), but a type I diabetic needs insulin.

271. The answer is D.

Apneusis can be described as an inspiratory cramp. Orthopnea is difficulty with breathing in a lying postion. Eupnea is normal breathing. Apnea is the absence of breathing.

272. The answer is B.

The pattern described in the question—a gradual increase in the rate and depth of respirations followed by periods of absent breathing—is known as Cheyne-Stokes breathing. Small breaths followed by inconsistent periods of absent breathing are known as a Biot's breathing pattern. Deep gasping breaths are known as a Kussmaul's breathing pattern. Awakening during the night due to periods of absent breathing is known as paroxysmal nocturnal dyspnea.

273. The answer is D.

This answer lists the stages of control in the correct order.

274. The answer is A.

These signs and symptoms are consistent with a lesion in the middle cerebral artery.

275. The answer is B.

This patient is likely to experience a decrease in the number of red blood cells. All of the other statements are correct. Fibrinogen drops initially but then rises throughout recovery.

276. The answer is C.

"Provide services for the length of time ordered" is not a summary of one of the principles of the code of ethics. If a physician orders an inappropriate frequency and/or duration, it is the responsibility of the therapist to resolve the dilemma to ensure that the patient is treated with an appropriate frequency and duration.

277. The answer is B.

This is a description of a dystrophic gait pattern, also called penguin gait. Patients with muscular dystrophy commonly demonstrate this gait pattern. A gluteus maximus gait presents with the patient leaning the trunk back while striking the heel on the involved side (or lurching). An arthrogenic gait pattern presents with the patient circumducting and elevating the hip on the involved side. This pattern is present with severe stiffness or a fused joint in the involved lower extremity. An antalgic gait pattern is exhibited when a person has pain with weight-bearing on the involved lower extremity.

278. The answer is C.

Residual volume, the amount of air left in the lungs after a forceful expiration, increases with age.

279. The answer is B.

Supine positioning after the first trimester is associated with decreased cardiac output.

280. The answer is C.

Although the patient will have to use the hemi-walker with the right upper extremity, answer C is still the best choice for this patient. Answers A and B are unsafe with one upper extremity. Answer D does not encourage weight-bearing and is not the most functional choice. A person with a cemented prosthesis can bear weight as tolerated on the involved lower extremity in early rehabilitation.

281. The answer is C.

The subjective complaints of "pins and needles" suggest that the source of the problem is either vascular or neurologic. Because thoracic outlet syndrome has been cleared, focus should be placed on the cervical spine.

282. The answer is D.

Answer D is the correct treatment. Strengthening is not indicated at this time, and splinting as described in answer C places too much stretch on the tendons. In addition, static splinting does not allow tendon gliding. Ultrasound is contraindicated over a healing tendon repair.

283. The answer is B.

This is the most appropriate response to a person who has not indicated that he or she has a medical background. If the patient's father inquires further, the therapist can be more detailed.

284. The answer is B.

The physical therapist can give his or her ideas about the treatment plan and possible functional outcomes after the evaluation. These ideas may change after treatment sessions and team meetings. The family should be continually informed of the patient's progress and expected level of function after discharge.

285. The answer is D.

The incentive spirometer provides visual feedback of maximal inspiratory efforts. The physical therapist is qualified to answer the patient's question.

286. The answer is D.

This patient has moderate lung disease. Because the intensity of exercise is low, frequency should increased to 5–7 times/week.

287. The answer is D.

Suctioning also can be performed in patients with significant hypoxemia.

288. The answer is D.

Answer A increases strength of the scalenes and sternocleidomastoid. Answer B strengthens the latissimus dorsi. Answer C increases the strength of the upper trapezius. All of these are accessory inspiratory muscles. Answer D strengthens the abdominals, which are muscles of forceful expiration.

289. The answer is D.

After the cross-bridge attaches to the thin filament (or actin), it moves, causing the thin filament to move. After the cross-bridge is broken, it moves into position to reattach to a thin filament (or actin) to repeat the cycle.

290. The answer is B.

These signs are characteristic of an arterial insufficiency ulcer. A venous ulcer often presents with the following symptoms: no pain around the wound, no gangrene, location typically on the medial ankle, pigmented skin around the ulcer, and significant edema. A trophic ulcer (also known as a pressure or decubitus ulcer) presents with decreased sensation, callused skin, and no pain and is located over bony prominences.

291. The answer is B.

Nursemaid's elbow is defined as dissociation of the radial head from the annular ligament. Choices A and D are usually due to a fall on an extended elbow. Erb's palsy is due to cervical trauma.

292. The answer is D.

This is an example of Russian stimulation.

293. The answer is D.

This is the most common placement suggested by sources used in preparation of this book. Spinal level varies, but the overall consensus is that the electrodes are placed higher and on the back initially. Then they are moved lower and to the anterior pubic region as labor progresses.

294. The answer is D.

This type of stimulation is usually not well tolerated by patients with acute conditions. Acute conditions are usually treated by TENS with a high frequency, and chronic conditions can be treated with a low frequency (if tolerated by the patient). Treatments providing a noxious stimulus usually have a longer-lasting effect.

295. The answer is A.

In Paget's disease (also known as osteitis deformans), bone is resorped and deposited at different rates during different stages of the disease. One of the deformities sometimes present is an enlarged cranium. This increased weight can result in compression fractures of the more superior cervical vertebrae. The origin of this condition is not exactly known. It usually involves people over 60 years of age.

296. The answer is B.

This patient is suffering from Guillain-Barré syndrome. Some permanent damage can result, with loss of sensory or motor function, but most patients make a full recovery in approximately 6 months. The syndrome often starts after a person has had a bout of the flu or a respiratory infection.

297. The answer is D.

This type of movement, known as athetosis, also can involve the feet, proximal parts of the extremities, and face. Chorea is rapid movements of the hands, wrist, or face. Ballism refers to forceful and uncontrollable throwing of the extremities outward. Lead-pipe rigidity is increasing resistance of an extremity to passive ranging. All of the above can result from damage to the basal ganglia.

298. The answer is C.

T-N-M is the most commonly recognized system of tumor staging. An Arabic number (0, 1, 2, or 3) follows each letter. The number behind the T represents the size of the tumor. Zero means no tumor. The higher the number, the larger the tumor. The number behind the N represents the degree of local lymph node involvement. Zero means no lymph node involvement. The higher the number, the greater the lymph node involvement. The number behind the M represents the degree of metastasis. Zero means no metastasis. The higher the number, the greater the degree of metastasis.

299. The answer is A.

Flexion and extension of the thumb are performed in a plane parallel to the palm of the hand. Abduction and adduction are performed in a plane perpendicular to the palm of the hand.

300. The answer is D.

The radial side is the lateral side of the forearm, which is innervated by the musculocutaneous nerve. The lateral antebrachial cutaneous nerve is a continuation of the musculocutaneous nerve.

301. The answer is D.

The right hemisphere is responsible for the left side of the body and vice versa. The limbs are at the top of the homunculus, the face is in the middle, and the organs are at the bottom.

302. The answer is A.

Adrenocorticotropic hormone, thyroid-stimulating hormone, growth hormone, follicle-stimulating hormone, and luteinizing hormone are all produced by the anterior pituitary gland. Insulin and glucagon are produced in the pancreas. Epinephrine and norepinephrine are produced in the adrenal medulla. Cortisol, androgens, and aldosterone are produced by the adrenal cortex.

303. The answer is D.

This patient has a lesion at the level of C7.

304. The answer is B.

The range considered "warm" for water settings in a whirlpool is between 35.5 and 36.5° Celsius, which is approximately 96–98° Fahrenheit. The formula for converting Celsius to Fahrenheit is F = (C × 9/5) + 32.

305. The answer is A.

The average adult wheelchair width is 26 inches, but the opening should be at least 32 inches to allow for hand clearance. A wheelchair ramp should be built with a 1:12 slope. The toilet seat needs to be between 17 and 19 inches in height.

306. The answer is D.

The therapist does not need to wear a gown, gloves, or mask. These precautions are necessary only if there is a chance that the therapist or his clothing can become contaminated with blood, serum, or feces.

307. The answer is C.

Mucoid sputum is clear or white and is not usually associated with infection. Thick sputum is referred to as tenacious. Foul-smelling sputum is called fetid and is often associated with infection.

308. The answer is B.

Frothy sputum is thin and white or has a slight pink color. This type of sputum is commonly present with pulmonary edema. Purulent sputum resembles pus, with a yellow or green color. Mucopurulent sputum is yellow to light green in color. Rusty sputum is a rust-colored sputum often associated with pneumonia.

309. The answer is B.

Yergason's test detects tendinitis of the long head of the biceps. Froment's sign is a test to determine adductor pollicis weakness due to ulnar nerve dysfunction. In the Waldron test, the patient performs squats while the therapist assesses the patella region for crepitus or pain. A positive test indicates possible chondromalacia. A positive Wilson test indicates possible osteochondritis dissecans. The test is performed by asking the patient to extend the knee in the seated position with internal rotation and again with external rotation of the tibia. The test is positive if there is pain with internal rotation and no pain with external rotation of the tibia.

310. The answer is C.

Increasing motor ability is not independent of motor learning. A therapist must facilitate motor learning with proper sensory cues and by promoting appropriate motor activity. Answer D is true because infants begin spontaneous movement, which later develops into more deliberate movement. Answer A is true because reflex movement can be used to develop more deliberate movement.

311. The answer is C.

The heart receives nerve impulses that travel through the sinoatrial node to the ventricles by way of the atrioventricular node, bundle branches, and Purkinje fibers.

312. The answer is D.

Acetic acid is sometimes used in attempts to dissolve a calcium deposit and is driven by the negative pole. Dexamethasone is an anti-inflammatory driven by the negative pole. Magnesium sulfate is used to decrease muscle spasms and is driven by the positive pole. Hydrocortisone is also used to treat inflammation and is driven by the positive pole.

313. The answer is A.

The popliteus, biceps femoris, and iliotibial band offer active restraint for the lateral side of the knee joint. The gastrocnemius assists in active restraint of the posterior side of the knee joint.

314. The answer is B.

In closed-chain activity, the femur medially rotates on the tibia. In open-chain activity, the tibia laterally rotates on the femur.

315. The answer is B.

The flexor digitorum profundus has four tendons, each attaching to the distal phalanx. If the three mentioned in the question are restricted, flexion at the distal interphalangeal joint in the normal hand would not be possible.

316. The answer is B.

The shrinker should be removed only for bathing. Because the surgical scars are healed, the stump can be immersed in water.

317. The answer is C.

This test assesses the strength of the latissimus dorsi. One of the functions of the latissimus is to push up from a sitting position. This test simulates that movement.

318. The answer is B.

Blisters should be allowed to subside naturally. Gel inserts lose their shape if not left in the prosthesis overnight. The prosthesis should be propped up in a corner or lain on the floor to prevent it from falling and cracking.

319. The answer is D.

All of the above are important skills for a patient with a hip disarticulation prosthesis to master, but posterior pelvic tilt should be mastered first to advance the prosthesis.

320. The answer is D.

Herpes zoster involves a particular dorsal root and its ganglia. TENS unit electrodes should be placed over the involved dermatome (L5 in this case).

321. The answer is A.

Because of poor balance, geriatric patients should increase the treadmill grade rather than the speed. Use of machines allows better posture and low intensities and limits the exercise within the patient's safe range of motion.

322. The answer is D.

Intermittent claudication is a sign of chronic arterial disease. Answer A is incorrect because it produces unilateral signs and symptoms. Answer B is incorrect because, although the signs and symptoms may be present in a patient with multiple sclerosis, this scenario paints a more accurate picture of a patient who has intermittent claudication. A compartment syndrome usually involves the anterior tibialis. In addition, patients with compartment syndrome require a longer rest time than this question implies before pain subsides.

323. The answer is A.

Hydrostatic (underwater) weighing involves comparing body weight in and out of water. Electrical impedance involves the principle that lean tissues have a greater electrolyte content than fat. Impedance measurements have a high margin of error. Anthropometric (skinfold) measurements also have a high margin of error, especially when made by unskilled individuals.

324. The answer is D.

Prone and sidelying positions would encourage flexion of the extremities with this patient. In this population, prone positioning allows more efficient cardiovascular function.

325. The answer is D.

Movements that stress the posterolateral hip joint capsule should be avoided. Sources vary on the exact amount of flexion that should be avoided. Passive hip abduction should be maintained after surgery with a wedge.

326. The answer is C.

A prolonged stretch assists in decreasing tone.

327. The answer is C.

To reach as described in the question, the patient must shift weight to the right buttock and elongate the right side of the trunk. With the same circumstances given in the question, but to the left side, the patient would shift weight to the left buttock and elongate the left side of the trunk.

328. The answer is A.

Isometric control develops before isotonic control.

329. The answer is A.

Avoiding the interossei helps to inhibit tone. Direct pressure to any hand musculature may increase tone. Hyperextension of the MCP joints also may cause an increase in tone.

330. The answer is C.

Deconditioned people benefit initially from low-intensity exercise with multiple sessions per day and per week.

331. The answer is C.

A tissue stretch end-feel is also felt with ankle dorsiflexion. An example of a bone-to-bone end-feel is with knee or elbow extension. Knee flexion is an example of soft tissue approximation. In an empty end-feel, a patient stops the movement due to pain.

332. The answer is D.

All of the following are capable of causing a noncapsular pattern.

333. The answer is D.

Sever's disease is traction apophysitis of the gastrocnemius tendon in children. In other words, the gastrocnemius attempts to pull away from the calcaneus, causing an inflammatory condition.

334. The answer is C.

No activity = 0. Slight contraction = 1+. Normal response = 2+. Exaggerated response = 3+. Severely exaggerated = 4+.

335. The answer is B.

When the test is performed on a patient with no motor neuron lesion, the umbilicus should move toward the stimulus. Unilateral movement suggests lower motor neuron involvement. A cremaster reflex is performed by stroking the medial thigh of a male with a sharp object. A normal response consists of superior movement of the scrotum on the ipsilateral side. An abnormal response is absence of scrotal movement on one side, which indicates possible lower motor neuron involvement. Bilateral absence of movement indicates upper motor neuron involvement.

336. The answer is D.

Meralgia paresthetica is the compression of the lateral femoral cutaneous nerve of the thigh as it passes under the inguinal ligament near the anterior superior iliac spine. Examples of the source of this problem include periods of obesity, postural changes, and tight clothing. Lumbar disc involvement and spondylolisthesis are less likely choices because the question indicates normal range of motion, lack of motor weakness, and no change with repeated active lumbar flexion.

337. The answer is A.

This patient most likely has a right anterior rotation of the right innominate and thus needs right posterior mobilization of the right innominate.

338. The answer is C.

This position, which limits inversion, plantar flexion, and adduction, is the most common position for ankle sprains.

339. The answer is A.

Bottle or breast feeding is rarely performed successfully before 34 weeks of gestational age. Sidelying position allows the infant to move the hands toward the mouth. The prone position encourages flexion. Full contact with the hand is more comforting to the infant.

340. The answer is D.

Although vibration often elicits a muscle contraction, a therapist should first choose stimuli that are more likely to occur naturally.

341. The answer is B.

Postural reactions are automatic unconscious reactions to changes in center of mass. Choice A is an appropriate goal but not always the most important.

342. The answer is A.

After the first 2 years of life, the femurs rotate to a more neutral position, and the amount of anteversion decreases.

343. The answer is C.

The signs and symptoms are most consistent with a slipped capital epiphysis. Bursitis presents with pain located over the bursa and is associated with overuse or rheumatoid arthritis. Avascular necrosis most frequently involves men 30–50 years of age. Septic arthritis is usually present in children 2 years of age or younger and often is due to steroid use or fever.

344. The answer is C.

Transverse (perpendicular to the scar) or circular massage assists in mobilization of scar tissue.

345. The answer is C.

Postural reactions and motor milestone development occur in the same sequence as with normal infants, but the progression of an infant with Down's syndrome is slower.

346. The answer is A.

The anterior cruciate ligament prevents excessive posterior roll of the femoral condyles during flexion of the femur at the knee joint.

347. The answer is D.

The ligament to which this question refers is the alar ligament. The tectorial membrane extends from the posterior part of C1 to the base of the occiput. The posterior atlanto-occipital ligament runs from the posterior arch of C1 to the posterior margin of the foramen magnum. The ligamentum nuchae is a triangular ligament that runs from the C7 spinous process to the external occipital protuberance.

348. The answer is A.

Patients with Parkinson's disease usually ambulate with the trunk in flexion. Increased trunk flexion causes a festinating gait to be more pronounced. Therapy should strengthen extensor muscles while stretching the flexors. Slow rocking has been shown to decrease tone, and biofeedback can improve a gait with shorter step and stride length by placement of markers on the floor for the feet.

349. The answer is B.

The anterior cruciate ligament is located within the articular cavity but outside the synovial lining. The anterior and posterior cruciate ligaments have their own synovial lining.

350. The answer is A.

These complaints are consistent with patellofemoral symptoms. The primary symptoms are pain in performing squats or ascending/descending stairs. Most patellofemoral pain is due to a lateral glide or tilt. This diagnosis is common in adolescent girls. Baker's cysts involve the posterior knee, and anterior cruciate ligament tears most often have a definite mechanism of injury.

351. The answer is A.

The patellofemoral joint is stressed less if exercised in the ranges noted in answer A, with open- and closed-chain exercises. Patellofemoral taping helps to decrease pain and therefore increases exercise participation. Answers B and C involve open-chain exercises that are performed within the range of 45–0 degrees of knee flexion.

352. The answer is B.

The patient is prone to excessive external rotation when attempting to extend the involved hip, because the gluteus minimus counteracts the lateral rotational force created by the gluteus maximus.

353. The answer is C.

The tests in choices A, B, and C assess the integrity of the anterior cruciate ligament. The pivot shift test is performed with the patient in supine position. The therapist applies a valgus stress with the lower leg internally rotated while passively flexing and extending the knee. A positive test is associated with instability with this motion. Lachman's test is similar to the anterior drawer test, but the knee is in slight flexion. In performing a posterior drawer test, the positioning is the same as for performing an anterior drawer test, but a posterior force is applied to the tibia to assess posterior cruciate ligament integrity. When performing these tests, the therapist is assessing the end-feel and amount of joint play to determine the integrity of the ligament.

354. The answer is C.

During pronation of the feet, the calcaneus everts, and the talus medially rotates and plantar flexes.

355. The answer is C.

At 1–2 weeks after surgery, the patient has an inflamed knee, and no functional testing can take place. Six weeks is an appropriate amount of time to allow inflammation to decrease enough for functional testing. Patients who have received a partial meniscectomy do not require as much healing time as patients who have received a meniscus repair.

356. The answer is B.

Plantar flexors have to contract in quiet standing. Other muscles are recruited with movement of the center of gravity.

357. The answer is A.

The talus is palpated just anterior and lateral to the medial malleolus. Supination is excessive lateral deviation of the talus, and pronation is excessive medial deviation.

358. The answer is A.

This is the primary function of the anterior inferior tibiofibular ligament.

359. The answer is B.

During a unilateral straight leg raise of the involved lower extremity, tension is placed on the sciatic nerve at approximately 35° of hip flexion. At 0° of hip flexion, tension is minimal to none, and tension is maximal above 70° of hip flexion.

360. The answer is B.

The patient has an extension lag, which may be due to any source that has inhibited the quadriceps and results in an inability to fully extend the knee actively.

361. The answer is D.

The posterior cruciate ligament becomes tight in full knee extension. This assists the tibia in external rotation, which is needed for the screw home mechanism with open-chain activities.

362. The answer is C.

Thompson's test checks the integrity of the Achilles' tendon. When this test is performed on an ankle with no dysfunction, squeezing the gastrocnemius causes passive plantar flexion of the ankle.

363. The answer is D.

When an exaggerated symmetrical tonic labyrinthine reflex is present, supine positioning increases extensor tone and prone positioning increases flexor tone. Sidelying also provides an opportunity for the physical therapist to stimulate flexion.

364. The answer is D.

The treatment techniques should be performed in the order of mobility, stability, controlled mobility, and skill.

365. The answer is A.

A valgus stress is most likely to injure any medial elbow structures, such as the ulnar nerve. The structures on the lateral side are likely to be injured with a varus stress. Choice C originates on the lateral supracondylar ridge.

366. The answer is B.

The extensor carpi radialis brevis absorbs most of the stress placed on the involved upper extremity in the position of wrist flexion, ulnar deviation, forearm pronation, and elbow extension (as with a backhand swing in tennis).

367. The answer is A.

Tennis elbow results from overuse of the wrist extensors. The shoulder external rotators should be used to power a backhand.

368. The answer is C.

The triangular fibrocartilage complex is made up of the dorsal radioulnar ligament, ulnar collateral ligament, ulnar articular cartilage, volar radioulnar ligament, ulnocarpal meniscus, and sheath of the extensor carpi ulnaris.

369. The answer is A.

Because the interossei cross the MP joints and the PIP joints, the PIP joints should be flexed with the MP joints in flexion and extension.

370. The answer is B.

The last position (3 inches) of the grip strength dynamometer tests the extrinsic muscles of the hand (muscles located in the forearm). The closer positions test the intrinsic muscles.

371. The answer is C.

Swan-neck deformity involves hyperextension of the proximal interphalangeal (PIP) joint and flexion of the distal interphalangeal (DIP) joint. Splinting to avoid this deformity is the treatment of choice. Boutonnière deformity involves flexion of the PIP joint and DIP joint hyperextension. Dupuytren's contracture is contracture of the palmar aponeurosis. Claw hand is the result of laceration of the ulnar nerve.

372. The answer is B.

The extensor carpi ulnaris is frequently subluxed after rupture of the triangular fibrocartilage complex. Subluxation leads to many mechanical changes in the wrist common in patients with rheumatoid arthritis.

373. The answer is C.

The radial pull component is designed to allow tightening of the radial side of the capsule.

374. The answer is D.

These signs and symptoms are common with median nerve compression as it travels through the two heads of the pronator teres. Carpal tunnel syndrome usually presents with a positive Tinel's sign, a positive Phalen's test, and decreased strength and sensation over the median nerve distribution. Ulnar nerve compression at Guyon's canal typically presents with numbness, pain, and tingling along the ulnar nerve distribution.

375. The answer is D.

This is the most stable position of the hip, which allows more normal growth.

376. The answer is D.

With a separation of this size, the therapist should use gentle abdominal strengthening while binding the abdominal region.

377. The answer is B.

Tarsal tunnel syndrome is caused by compression of the posterior tibial nerve as it travels through the tarsal tunnel. The tarsal tunnel is formed by the medial malleolus, medial collateral ligament, talus, and calcaneus.

378. The answer is A.

Normally, the ankle requires 20° or more of dorsiflexion for a patient to run or ascend/descend stairs properly. Independent ambulation with a normal gait pattern requires 10° of dorsiflexion.

379. The answer is D.

Because of the length of the time since the surgical procedure, the patient may have adhesive capsulitis. The capsule should continue to be stretched to increase range of motion. The patient should visit the physician if the range-of-motion deficits continue.

380. The answer is D.

Both anaerobic and aerobic systems are active during rest. The anaerobic system is working at least at a cellular level during rest. The level of lactic acid produced at rest is not enough to cause any build-up. The aerobic system is also working at least at a cellular level during high-intensity activity.

381. The answer is D.

The muscle spindles are responsible for the stretch reflex. When a muscle is stretched too quickly, the muscle spindles cause the muscle to contract and shorten (which is called the stretch reflex). The Golgi tendon organs are responsible for the inverse stretch reflex. They are located in the junction between the muscle and tendon and detect changes in tension. When a tendon is stretched too quickly, the Golgi tendon organs cause the muscle to relax.

382. The answer is C.

Because the scaphoid has a poor vascular supply, aggressive therapy should be avoided until the bone is fully healed (12–24 weeks). A Colles' fracture (fracture of the distal radius with dorsal movement of the fixed segment) should heal in 6–8 weeks. A boxer's fracture (fracture of the fifth metacarpal) requires 4–6 weeks. A Bennett's fracture (fracture of the proximal first metacarpal) usually requires 6–8 weeks. The length of healing time given in the above examples obviously depends on the individual patient and the type of surgical fixation (if any).

383. The answer is A.

The patient has an irritation of the iliotibial band as it passes over the lateral femoral epicondyle. This occurs at approximately 30° from full knee extension.

384. The answer is A.

When the hindfoot is pronated, the forefoot (transverse tarsal joints) can compensate for uneven terrain. If the hindfoot is supinated, the forefoot also is likely to supinate and possibly cause damage to the lateral ankle ligaments.

385. The answer is A.

Lateral step-ups are probably too difficult for a patient who received an anterior ligament reconstruction with a patella tendon autograft 2 weeks ago.

386. The answer is C.

The wrists should be in neutral position when the fingers are on the middle row of the keyboard.

387. The answer is C.

Tools with small handles require more grip strength. Tasks below shoulder height reduce the risk of impingement, and more force can be applied to tasks if they are kept below elbow height.

388. The answer is B.

Learning wheelchair safety techniques would be difficult for this patient in this stage of recovery, who have a difficult time learning new skills (because they are confused and easily agitated). Treatment should include activities that are familiar to the patient.

389. The answer is D.

The Golgi tendon organs monitor tension at the musclotendonous junction. Ruffini endings are located in the joint capsule, ligaments, and deep layers of the dermis. Meissner's corpuscles are located in the dermis. Merkel's disks are located below the epidermis.

390. The answer is A.

In response to a pronated subtalar joint, the forefoot undergoes a supination twist and the first ray dorsiflexes. Because the distal first cuneiform is convex and the proximal first metatarsal is concave, inferior mobilization of the first metatarsal is required.

391. The answer is D.

A patient with severe knee flexion contractures has a line of gravity that is anterior to the hip, posterior to the knee, and anterior to the ankle. This causes a flexion moment at the hip, knee, and ankle.

392. The answer is D.

A patient with hammer toes exhibits hyperextension of the distal interphalangeal joints and metatarsophalangeal joints and flexion of the proximal interphalangeal joints.

393. The answer is B.

To maintain balance, the lumbar spine must laterally flex toward the supporting lower extremity during single-limb support.

394. The answer is D.

Choice D is the length of stride during one gait cycle. Choice A describes a decreased step length, choice B describes a decrease in step duration, and choice C describes a decrease in single-limb support time.

395. The answer is A.

The tibialis anterior, extensor digitorum longus, and extensor hallucis longus contract concentrically to achieve a neutral ankle position before initial contact.

396. The answer is C.

The right shoulder and thorax begin to move forward at heel strike (initial contact).

397. The answer is A.

The hamstrings bring the knee to approximately 60° of flexion during acceleration. The hip flexors, ankle dorsiflexors, and toe extensors are also active.

398. The answer is C.

The geriatric population would have a longer period of double support in an attempt to maintain balance. They also would have a shorter step and stride length.

399. The answer is D.

A warm whirlpool with the lower extremity in a dependent position is likely to increase the edema. An Unna boot is cotton gauze covered with zinc oxide, gelatin, and calamine. It is put on much like an ACE wrap. The boot is left to harden overnight, and the dressing resists further edema because of its rigidity. A compression pump is often used for increased edema in the extremities.

400. The answer is A.

A heel that is too stiff causes excessive knee flexion. Choices B and C cause excessive knee extension during this stage of the gait cycle.

BIBLIOGRAPHY

1. Agur AMR: Grant's Atlas of Anatomy, 9th ed. Baltimore, Williams & Wilkins, 1991.
2. Brooks DS: Program Design for Personal Trainers: Bridging Theory into Application. Champaign, IL, Human Kinetics, 19978.
3. Charness A, Schneider FJ: Stroke/Head Injury: A Guide to Functional Outcomes in Physical Therapy Management. Gaithersburg, MD, Aspen Publishers, 1986.
4. Ciccone CD: Pharmacology in Rehabilitation. Philadelphia, F.A. Davis, 1996.
5. Connolly BH, Montgomery PO: Therapeutic Exercise in Developmental Disabilities, 2nd ed. Hixson, TN, Chattanooga Group, 1993.
6. Elston RC, Johnson WD: Essentials of Biostatistics, 2nd ed. Philadelphia, F.A. Davis, 1994.
7. Hayes KW: Manual for Physical Agents, 4th ed. Norwalk, CT, Appleton & Lange, 1993.
8. Hillegass EA, Sadowsky HS: Essentials of Cardiopulmonary Physical Therapy. Philadelphia, W.B. Saunders, 1994.
9. Hoppenfeld S: Physical Examination of the Spine and Extremities. Norwalk, CT, Appleton & Lange, 1976.
10. Jenkins DB: Hollinshead's Functional Anatomy of the Limbs and Back, 6th ed. Philadelphia, W.B. Saunders, 1991.
11. Karacoloff LA, Hammersley CS, Schneider FJ: Lower Extremity Amputation, 2nd ed. Gaithersburg, MD, Aspen Publishers, 1992.
12. Kenney WL, Humphrey RH, Bryant CX: ASCM's Guidelines for Exercise Testing and Prescription, 5th ed. Baltimore, Williams & Wilkins, 1995.
13. Kettenbach G: Writing Soap Notes, 2nd ed. Philadelphia, F.A. Davis, 1995.
14. Kisner C, Colby LA: Therapeutic Exercise: Foundations and Techniques. Philadelphia, F.A. Davis, 1990.
15. Liebler JG, Levine RE, Rothman J: Management Principles for Health Professionals, 2nd ed. Gaithersburg, MD, Aspen Publishers, 1992.
16. Magee DJ: Orthopedic Physical Assessment, 2nd ed. Philadelphia, W.B. Saunders, 1992.
17. Minor MA, Minor SD: Patient Care Skills, 2nd ed. Norwalk, CT, Appleton & Lange, 1990.
18. Minor MA, Minor SD: Patient Care Skills, 3rd ed. Norwalk, CT, Appleton & Lange, 1995.
19. Michlovitz SL: Thermal Agents in Rehabilitation, 2nd ed. Philadelphia, F.A. Davis, 1990.
20. Michlovitz SL: Thermal Agents in Rehabilitation, 3rd ed. Philadelphia, F.A. Davis, 1996.
21. Netter FH: Atlas of Human Anatomy. Summit, NJ, Ciba-Geigy Corporation, 1989.
22. Noback CR, Strominger NL, Demarest RJ: The Human Nervous System, 4th ed. Philadelphia, Lea & Febiger, 1991.
23. Norkin CC, Levangie PK: Joint Structure and Function, 2nd ed. Philadelphia, F.A. Davis, 1992.
24. Norkin CC, White DJ: Measurement of Joint Motion, 2nd ed. Philadelphia, F.A. Davis, 1995.
25. Novak TJ, Handford AG: Essentials of Pathophysiology. Dubuque, IA, William C. Brown, 1994.
26. Montgomery PC, Connolly BH: Motor Control and Physical Therapy, 2nd ed. Hixson, TN, Chattanooga Group, 1995.
27. O'Sullivan SB, Schmitz TJ: Physical Rehabilitation Assessment and Treatment, 3rd ed. Philadelphia, F.A. Davis, 1994.
28. Pedretti LW: Occupational Therapy: Practice Skills for Physical Dysfunction, 2nd ed. St. Louis, Mosby, 1985.
29. Rancho Los Amigos Medical Center: Observational Gait Analysis. Rancho Los Amigos Medical Center, Downy, CA, 1993.
30. Richardson JK, Iglarsh ZA: Clinical Orthopedic, Physical Therapy, Philadelphia, W.B. Saunders, 1994.
31. Robinson AJ, Synder-Mackler L: Clinical Electrophysiology, 2nd ed. Baltimore, Williams & Wilkins, 1995.
32. Rothstein JM, Roy SH, Wolf SL: The Rehabilitation Specialist Handbook. Philadelphia, F.A. Davis, 1991.
33. Scully RM, Barnes MR: Physical Therapy. Philadelphia, J.B. Lippincott, 1989.
34. Starkey C: Therapeutic Modalities for Athletic Trainers. Philadelphia, F.A. Davis, 1993.
35. Sullivan PE, Markos PD: Clinical Decision Making in Therapeutic Exercise. Norwalk, CT, Appleton & Lange, 1995.
36. Summers MF: Spinal Cord Injury. Norwalk, CT, Appleton & Lange, 1992.
37. Thomas CL: Taber's Cyclopedic Medical Dictionary, 17th ed. Philadelphia, F.A. Davis, 1989.
38. Vander AJ, Sherman JH, Luciano DS: Human Physiology: The Mechanism of Body Function, New York, McGraw-Hill, 1994.
39. Williams SJ, Torrens PR: Introduction to Health Sciences, 4th ed. Albany, NY, Delmar Publishers, 1993.